Differential Diagnosis of Chest Pain

Edited by Umashankar Lakshmanadoss

Published in London, United Kingdom

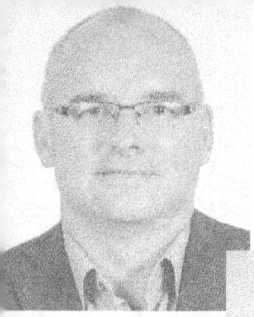
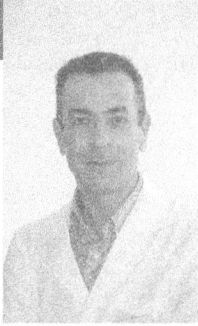
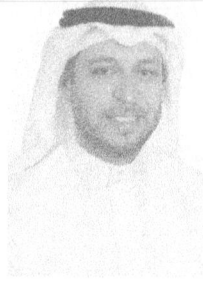
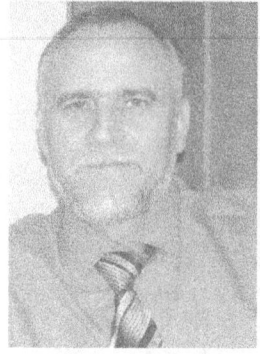
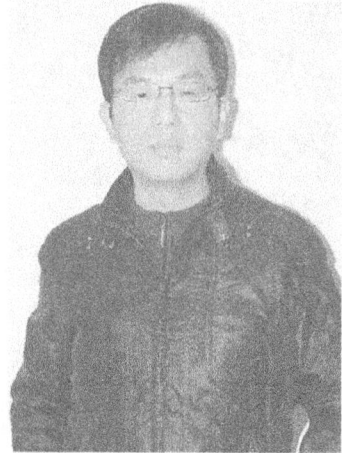
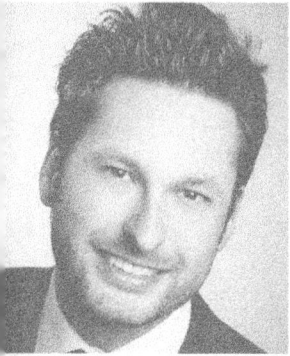
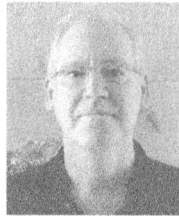

IntechOpen

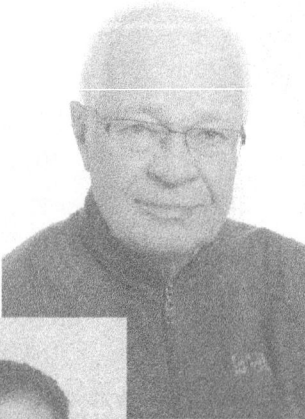
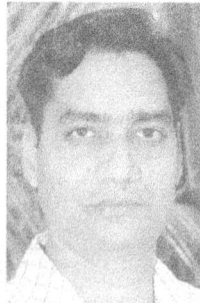
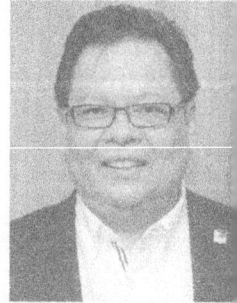
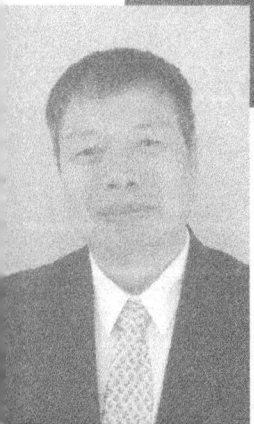
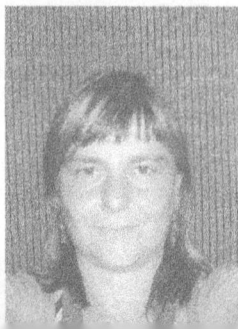
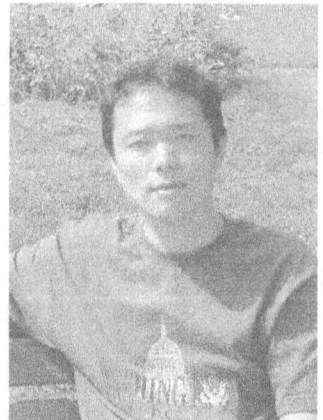

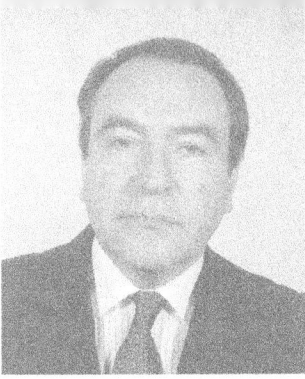

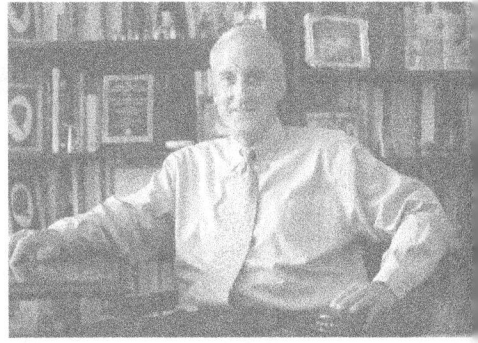

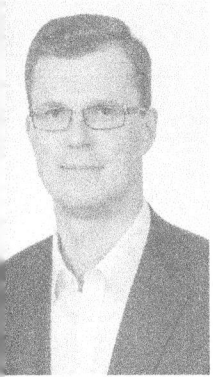

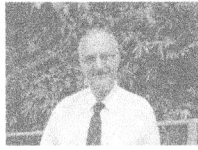

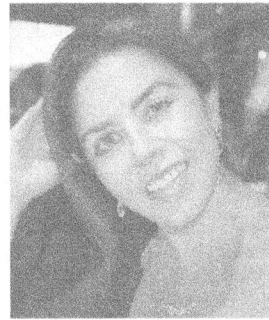

Supporting open minds since 2005

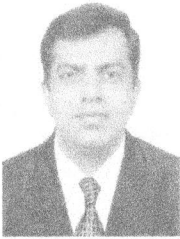

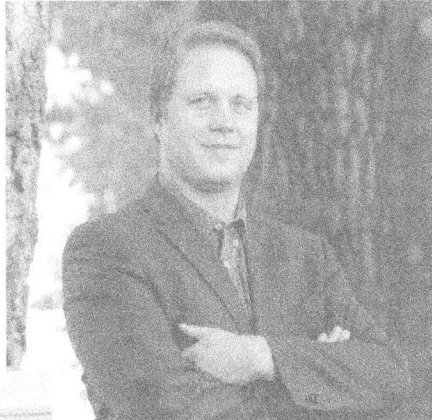

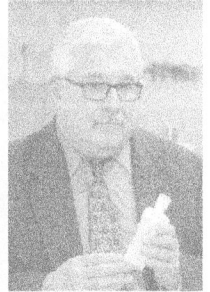

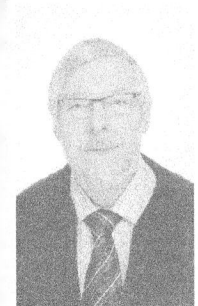

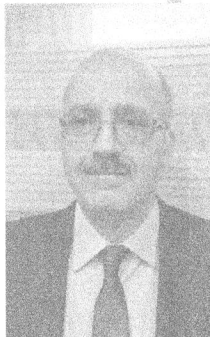

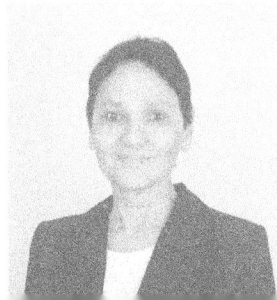

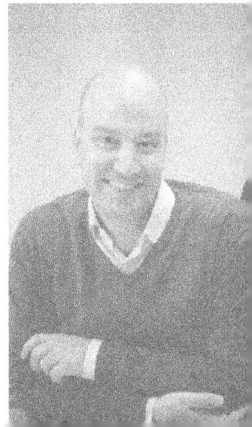

Differential Diagnosis of Chest Pain
http://dx.doi.org/10.5772/intechopen.78875
Edited by Umashankar Lakshmanadoss

Contributors
Ghulam Naroo, Bina Nasim, Mohammad Anas, Sardar Zafar, Laji Mathew, Ahmed Sajjad, Anis Shaikh, John-Ross Clarke, Gilead Lancaster, Mehmet Semih Demirtas, Umashankar Lakshmanadoss, Karnika Senthilkumar, Imran Sulemankhil, Nikolaos Koumallos, Michael Demosthenous, Konstantinos Triantafyllou

Notice
Statements and opinions expressed in the chapters are these of the individual contributors and not necessarily those of the editors or publisher. No responsibility is accepted for the accuracy of information contained in the published chapters. The publisher assumes no responsibility for any damage or injury to persons or property arising out of the use of any materials, instructions, methods or ideas contained in the book.

First published in London, United Kingdom, 2020 by IntechOpen
IntechOpen is the global imprint of INTECHOPEN LIMITED, registered in England and Wales, registration number: 11086078, 7th floor, 10 Lower Thames Street, London,
EC3R 6AF, United Kingdom
Printed in Croatia

British Library Cataloguing-in-Publication Data
A catalogue record for this book is available from the British Library

Additional hard and PDF copies can be obtained from orders@intechopen.com

Differential Diagnosis of Chest Pain
Edited by Umashankar Lakshmanadoss
p. cm.
Print ISBN 978-1-83880-589-0
Online ISBN 978-1-83880-590-6
eBook (PDF) ISBN 978-1-83880-591-3

We are IntechOpen,
the world's leading publisher of
Open Access books
Built by scientists, for scientists

4,900+
Open access books available

123,000+
International authors and editors

140M+
Downloads

Our authors are among the

151
Countries delivered to

Top 1%
most cited scientists

12.2%
Contributors from top 500 universities

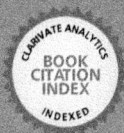

Interested in publishing with us?
Contact book.department@intechopen.com

Numbers displayed above are based on latest data collected.
For more information visit www.intechopen.com

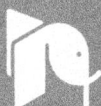

Meet the editor

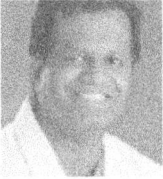

Dr. Umashankar Lakshmanadoss completed his training from the University of Rochester, NY, USA. He served as Director of Inpatient Medical Consult Service at Johns Hopkins University School of Medicine and then joined the Division of Cardiovascular Medicine at Guthrie Clinic, Sayre, PA, USA. Then he pursued training in cardiac electrophysiology at William Beaumont School of Medicine and continued advanced cardiac electrophysiology training at Mayo Clinic, Rochester, MN. He served as an Assistant Professor of Medicine in the Division of Cardiology, Louisiana State University, Shreveport, LA, where he also serves as the Director of Complex Arrhythmia Ablation Program. His research interest is in the field of cardiac electrophysiology. Currently, he is the Director of Cardiac Electrophysiology at Mercy Health, Cincinnati, USA.

Contents

Preface

Cardiovascular disease continues to be the leading cause of morbidity and mortality in both developed and developing countries. Chest pain is one of the common and distressing presentations of cardiovascular disease. The number of patients presenting to emergency rooms or to their healthcare providers with chest pain is ever-growing and constitutes one of the most common reasons to seek medical help. Out of these patients with chest pain, cardiovascular cause constitutes about 20% of the patients, and out of which only 5% is a truly acute life-threatening disease. Hence, it is very important to have a systematic approach to patients with chest pain. The clinical scenario is the most important factor to differentiate the various causes of chest pain so that these patients can be treated at the earliest to avoid a bad outcome. It also vital to diagnose non acute/non cardiac chest pains and decipher their etiology as these patients could be frequently visiting the health care providers without a proper diagnosis.

This book aims to provide an excellent overview of the differential diagnosis and approach to chest pain in various clinical settings. This book is divided into two sections including the introduction and approach to chest pain. Our introductory chapter starts with the basic principles of statistics and its application in various diagnostic modalities of heart disease. Our authors present a nice approach to patients presenting with chest pain in various scenarios. We have also included a chapter describing GERD, which could present as chest pain and another chapter describing aortic dissection, which is a life-threatening disease presenting with chest pain. We hope that this book will serve as an accessible handbook on differential diagnosis of chest pain.

I gratefully acknowledge the invaluable organizational skills of the publisher IntechOpen, timely, patient and invaluable assistance of Author Service Manager Ms. Dolores Kuzelj, designer, technical generators, information technology staff and finally the marketing representatives who are working constantly to promote the book on various platforms. I sincerely appreciate and applaud all the contributing authors for their excellence, hard work and commitment to the chapters. They have taken time from their personal and professional lives to complete this task. I thank them profusely for that.

This book is dedicated to my son Shawn who continues to inspire me, making my life blissful and giving me the confidence that every generation is better than the one before.

Umashankar Lakshmanadoss MD, CCDS, FHRS
Mercy Heart Institute,
Cincinnati, OH, USA

Section 1

Introduction

Chapter 1

Introductory Chapter: The Patient Presenting with Chest Pain

John-Ross D. Clarke

1. Background

Chest pain is the principal reason for approximately 5% of the emergency department (ED) visits in the United States [1]. It is the most frequent reason for presentation to an emergency facility in men age 65 years and older. In some cohorts, chest pain accounts for up to 16% of ambulance transports and constitutes almost 30% of emergency admissions [2, 3]. In the primary care setting however, less than 1% of visits are for a chief complaint of chest pain [4].

Part of the significance of chest pain as a presenting symptom is its association with potentially life-threatening diagnoses such as: acute myocardial infarction (AMI), pulmonary embolism, and aortic dissection, among others. The challenge for the clinician is the accurate stratification of patients based on risk, and the efficient and cost-effective utilization of resources to establish a diagnosis. The first step in diagnosis is an informed history and physical examination- which is not without limitations even in the most experienced hands [5]. The sections that follow provide a brief insight into the scope of chest pain diagnoses and the value of clinical findings in establishing a diagnosis.

2. The differential diagnosis of chest pain

The differential diagnosis of a patient presenting with chest pain is extensive [6]. A systematic approach is therefore needed to (i) determine the likelihood of an immediately life-threatening cause, (ii) differentiate cardiac from noncardiac etiologies, and (iii) reduce over-diagnosis and thus overutilization of healthcare resources in the subsequent investigation. This approach not only increases the diagnostic accuracy and efficiency of workup, but also leads to better patient and clinician satisfaction [7].

There are innumerable ways of categorizing the differential diagnosis of chest pain. Potential categorization approaches are: (i) cardiac vs. noncardiac etiologies (ii) classifying based on symptom characteristics, (iii) by organ systems and (iv) anatomically (**Figure 1**). An anatomic approach allows for an exhaustive differential diagnosis but does have limitations in refinement based on pre-test probability- this subsequent step requires the incorporation of other aspects of symptom presentation [6].

A schema for classifying causes of chest pain anatomically includes structures from the skin to internal organs of the thorax and upper abdomen (**Figure 1**).

3

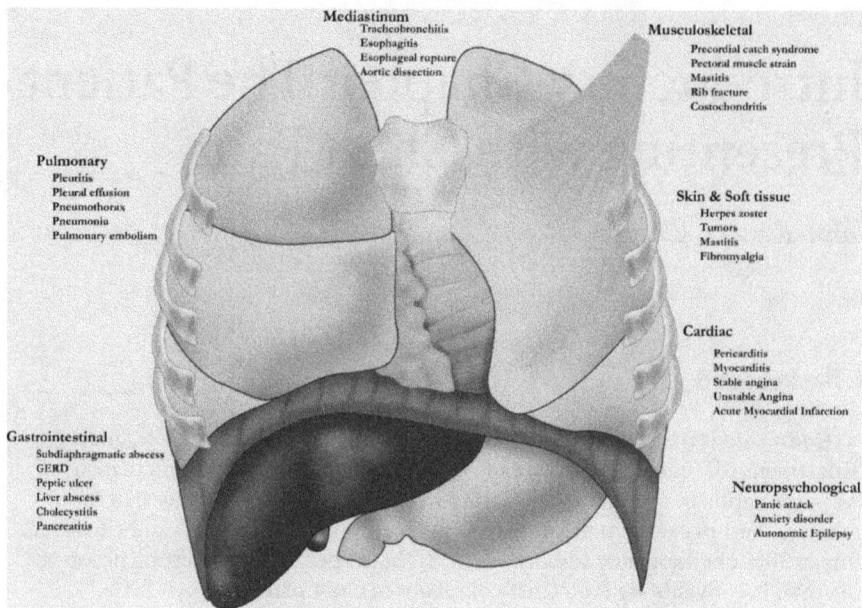

Figure 1.
An anatomic approach to the differential diagnosis of chest pain.

3. The clinical value of the chest pain presentation

The clinical assessment of a patient presenting with chest pain has undergone extensive research, particularly in its ability to detect ischemic cardiac and other life-threatening causes, e.g., acute pulmonary embolism [5]. Due to the potential limitations of history and physical examination in certain settings, the inclusion of early diagnostic tools such as the electrocardiogram, or serum d-dimer, have been validated in many risk prediction models to aid the clinician in decision making [8].

In addition to the details of the chest pain history, the acuity and setting of patient presentation also provide valuable clues to the differential. The traditional life-threatening conditions taught in medical training have been found to make up about 5% of the chest pain diagnoses in ED visits [9]. Over 90% of these life-threatening diagnoses are due to acute coronary syndrome (ACS). In the primary care setting on the contrary, less than 2% of patients will end up having ACS [10]. Up to one-third of the causes for chest pain in ambulatory visits are due to chest wall-related pain [11, 12].

All the important considerations of chest pain details will not be covered here. Key qualifiers though are the location, quality, acuity, evolution, and the frequency of the pain; as well as a history of prior ischemic cardiac events (of similar or differing character). Additional information is needed on associated symptoms as well as aggravating and relieving factors [13]. This large volume of data can be synthesized into illness scripts to describe the most likely syndrome(s) accounting for the chest pain. This summative processing allows for further diagnostic refinement, especially when discordant information is present [14].

It is worth reiterating that the art of history taking is susceptible to misinterpretation on the part of both the interviewer and the patient. Cognitive biases from the clinician and cultural differences in the understanding of certain descriptors means that interpretations should be restated and clarified throughout the history taking process [15].

3.1 Diagnostic accuracy of symptoms and signs in acute coronary syndromes

No single clinical symptom or sign can rule in or out the possibility of ACS or acute MI. However, a constellation of patient characteristics, clinical symptoms and signs can be used to determine the pretest likelihood with some diagnostic accuracy [16]. The traditional highest risk group has been patients of male gender, older than 60 years, presenting with "pressure-type" chest pain radiating to the neck, shoulder or arm [17].

The traditional predictor of "pressure-like" symptoms has been noted to have only a likelihood ratio of between 1 and 2 in predicting AMI in patients presenting with chest pain. The use of "sharp" or "stabbing" to characterize symptoms more significantly decreases the likelihood of MI (LR− = 0.3) [18]. Descriptors associated with the diagnosis of AMI in decreasing order of likelihood are: (i) pain radiating to the right and left arm simultaneously (LR+ = 7.1), (ii) association with exertion (LR+ = 2.4), (iii) radiation to the left arm only (LR+ = 2.3) and (iv) association with diaphoresis (LR+ = 2.0). Conversely, symptoms associated with increasing likelihood of the pain not being related to AMI are: (i) absence of an relation to exertion (LR− = 0.8) and (ii) descriptors such as "pleuritic" or "positional variation" (LR− = 0.2 & 0.3 respectively) [5].

3.2 Diagnostic accuracy of symptoms and signs in noncardiac causes of chest pain

Once a cardiac etiology of chest pain is deemed to be unlikely, the diagnostic puzzle is in determining which of the many other differentials is most likely. Fortunately, similar to their cardiac counterparts, noncardiac etiologies have certain key features on both history of physical exam which can be used to streamline the diagnostic approach.

It was mentioned earlier that chest wall-related pain is the most common etiology in some ambulatory settings. Four clinical symptoms/signs which are highly suggestive of a chest wall-related etiology are: localized muscle tension, "stinging" nature of the pain, reproducibility on palpation and an absence of cough [16]. The presence of at least two of these findings has a LR+ of 3.0.

No evidence-based clinical maneuvers exist to aid in the diagnosis of gastro-esophageal reflux disease (GERD) [10]. Common associated complaints are "burning" retrosternal discomfort, regurgitation of gastric contents and a bitter taste in the mouth [19]. One approach which is supported by evidence, is the response of symptoms to a one-week trial of proton pump inhibitors (LR+ = 3.1; LR− = 0.3) [20].

Other less common causes of chest pain such as pneumonia, pulmonary embolism and acute thoracic dissection can be suspected based on history but cannot be ruled in or out without the support of definitive testing. Features such as fever, cough and pleurisy (with suggestive examination findings), have a performance of LR+ = 2.0; LR− = 0.24 for the diagnosis of pneumonia [21]. Validated clinical decision tools, such as Well's criteria, guide further testing when a pulmonary embolism is suspected [22]. Finally, although acute chest pain and/or back pain with an upper extremity pulse differential can help with risk stratification for the likelihood of an acute thoracic aortic dissection (LR+ = 5.3), definitive imaging is required [23].

4. Outcomes and implications of patients presenting with chest pain

Half of the chest pain presentations to the ED are left unspecified [9]. The majority of these end up being noncardiac etiologies when they are followed up in the primary care setting. In patients presenting to the ambulatory setting for the first time with chest pain, etiologies such as angina, AMI, musculoskeletal pain or GERD can be diagnosed at the first consultation. However, the incidence of chest pain going unspecified remains about 15 per 1000 person-years [24]. Approximately 2–10% of these individuals will go on to have cardiovascular disease as the cause of their symptoms [25]. A definitive diagnosis is most often made by 12 weeks of follow-up- if not within the first year. During this time period though, patients are likely to have: (i) seen their physician on up to three separate occasions, (ii) been referred to a specialist or (iii) hospitalized [24]. This time course leads to both clinician and patient anxiety, and can negatively impact quality of life [26].

One of the feared outcomes in patients presenting to an ED with chest pain, is the inadvertent discharge of someone with ACS. Older estimates suggested rates of this could be as high as 2% [27]. Thankfully, with the advent of newer diagnostic modalities, risk scores and investigative protocols, the risk of this outcome is likely to continue to decline [28]. An effort to mitigate this risk must be balanced against the costly and potentially harmful consequences of unnecessary hospitalization or extensive workup [28]. The fear of missing a potentially life-threatening diagnosis like ACS is no less apparent with ambulatory contact [29].

5. Conclusions

Chest pain is a common reason for hospital admission. Most patients who present to either an emergency department or primary care clinic will end up having a noncardiac cause of their symptoms. However, due to the poor outcomes associated with cardiovascular etiologies, significant healthcare resources are used in ruling in or out ischemic cardiac causes; when an alternative is not obvious. For these reasons, it is prudent that we continue to develop systems to efficiently differentiate between the many causes of chest pain.

Conflict of interest

The author has no conflicts of interest to declare.

Author details

John-Ross D. Clarke
Department of Internal Medicine, Yale-New Haven Health Bridgeport Hospital, Bridgeport, CT, USA

*Address all correspondence to: johnrossclarke@gmail.com

IntechOpen

References

[1] Rui P, Kang K, Ashman JJ. National Hospital Ambulatory Medical Care Survey: 2016 emergency department summary tables. 2016. https://www.cdc.gov/nchs/data/ahcd/nhamcs_emergency/2016_ed_web_tables.pdf [Accessed: 07 February 2020]

[2] Pedersen CK, Stengaard C, Friesgaard K, Dodt KK, Sondergaard HM, Terkelsen CJ, et al. Chest pain in the ambulance; prevalence, causes and outcome—A retrospective cohort study. Scandinavian Journal of Trauma, Resuscitation and Emergency Medicine. 2019;**27**(1):84

[3] Goodacre S, Cross E, Arnold J, Angelini K, Capewell S, Nicholl J. The health care burden of acute chest pain. Heart. 2005;**91**(2):229-230

[4] Hsiao CJ, Cherry DK, Beatty PC, Rechtsteiner EA. National Ambulatory Medical Care Survey: 2007 summary. National Health Statistics Report. 2010;**3**(27):1-32

[5] Swap CJ, Nagurney JT. Value and limitations of chest pain history in the evaluation of patients with suspected acute coronary syndromes. JAMA. 2005;**294**(20):2623-2629

[6] Stern SDC, Cifu AS, Altkorn D. Chest pain. In: Symptom to Diagnosis: An Evidence-Based Guide. United States: McGraw-Hill Education/Medical; 2014

[7] Gigerenzer G. Reckoning with Risk: Learning to Live with Uncertainty. Penguin Books Limited; 2003

[8] Wells PS, Anderson DR, Rodger M, Ginsberg JS, Kearon C, Gent M, et al. Derivation of a simple clinical model to categorize patients probability of pulmonary embolism: Increasing the models utility with the SimpliRED D-dimer. Thrombosis and Haemostasis. 2000;**83**(3):416-420

[9] Hsia RY, Hale Z, Tabas JA. A national study of the prevalence of life-threatening diagnoses in patients with chest pain. JAMA Internal Medicine. 2016;**176**(7):1029-1032

[10] McConaghy JR, Oza RS. Outpatient diagnosis of acute chest pain in adults. American Family Physician. 2013;**87**(3):177-182

[11] Klinkman MS, Stevens D, Gorenflo DW. Episodes of care for chest pain: A preliminary report from MIRNET Michigan research network. Journal of Family Practice. 1994;**38**(4):345-352

[12] Haasenritter J, Biroga T, Keunecke C, Becker A, Donner-Banzhoff N, Dornieden K, et al. Causes of chest pain in primary care—A systematic review and meta-analysis. Croatian Medical Journal. 2015;**56**(5):422-430

[13] Morrow DA. Chest discomfort. In: Harrison's Principles of Internal Medicine. McGraw-Hill Education/Medical; 2017

[14] Wheeler DJ, Cascino T, Sharpe BA, Connor DM. When the script doesn't fit: An exercise in clinical reasoning. Journal of General Internal Medicine. 2017;**32**(7):836-840

[15] Summers RL, Cooper GJ, Carlton FB, Andrews ME, Kolb JC. Prevalence of atypical chest pain descriptions in a population from the southern United States. American Journal of the Medical Sciences. 1999;**318**(3):142-145

[16] Bosner S, Becker A, Abu Hani M, Keller H, Sonnichsen AC, Haasenritter J, et al. Accuracy of symptoms and signs for coronary heart disease assessed in primary care. British Journal of General Practice. 2010;**60**(575):e246-e257

[17] Rouan GW, Lee TH, Cook EF, Brand DA, Weisberg MC, Goldman L. Clinical characteristics and outcome of acute myocardial infarction in patients with initially normal or nonspecific electrocardiograms (a report from the Multicenter chest pain study). The American Journal of Cardiology. 1989;**64**(18):1087-1092

[18] Panju AA, Hemmelgarn BR, Guyatt GH, Simel DL. The rational clinical examination. Is this patient having a myocardial infarction? JAMA. 1998;**280**(14):1256-1263

[19] Zimmerman J. Validation of a brief inventory for diagnosis and monitoring of symptomatic gastro-oesophageal reflux. Scandinavian Journal of Gastroenterology. 2004;**39**(3):212-216

[20] Wang WH, Huang JQ, Zheng GF, Wong WM, Lam SK, Karlberg J, et al. Is proton pump inhibitor testing an effective approach to diagnose gastroesophageal reflux disease in patients with noncardiac chest pain?: A meta-analysis. Archives of Internal Medicine. 2005;**165**(11):1222-1228

[21] Diehr P, Wood RW, Bushyhead J, Krueger L, Wolcott B, Tompkins RK. Prediction of pneumonia in outpatients with acute cough—A statistical approach. Journal of Chronic Diseases. 1984;**37**(3):215-225

[22] Wells PS, Anderson DR, Rodger M, Stiell I, Dreyer JF, Barnes D, et al. Excluding pulmonary embolism at the bedside without diagnostic imaging: Management of patients with suspected pulmonary embolism presenting to the emergency department by using a simple clinical model and d-dimer. Annals of Internal Medicine. 2001;**135**(2):98-107

[23] von Kodolitsch Y, Schwartz AG, Nienaber CA. Clinical prediction of acute aortic dissection. Archives of Internal Medicine. 2000;**160**(19):2977-2982

[24] Ruigomez A, Rodriguez LA, Wallander MA, Johansson S, Jones R. Chest pain in general practice: Incidence, comorbidity and mortality. Family Practice. 2006;**23**(2):167-174

[25] Robson J, Ayerbe L, Mathur R, Addo J, Wragg A. Clinical value of chest pain presentation and prodromes on the assessment of cardiovascular disease: A cohort study. BMJ Open. 2015;**5**(4):e007251

[26] Eslick GD. Noncardiac chest pain: Epidemiology, natural history, health care seeking, and quality of life. Gastroenterology Clinics of North America. 2004;**33**(1):1-23

[27] Pope JH, Aufderheide TP, Ruthazer R, Woolard RH, Feldman JA, Beshansky JR, et al. Missed diagnoses of acute cardiac ischemia in the emergency department. New England Journal of Medicine. 2000;**342**(16):1163-1170

[28] Amsterdam EA, Kirk JD, Bluemke DA, Diercks D, Farkouh ME, Garvey JL, et al. Testing of low-risk patients presenting to the emergency department with chest pain: A scientific statement from the American Heart Association. Circulation. 2010;**122**(17):1756-1776

[29] Hoorweg BB, Willemsen RT, Cleef LE, Boogaerts T, Buntinx F, Glatz JF, et al. Frequency of chest pain in primary care, diagnostic tests performed and final diagnoses. Heart. 2017;**103**(21):1727-1732

Section 2

Approach to Chest Pain

Chapter 2

Application of Bayesian Principles to the Evaluation of Coronary Artery Disease in the Modern Era

John-Ross D. Clarke and Gilead I. Lancaster

Abstract

The number of testing modalities available for the diagnosis of significant coronary artery disease has grown over the last few decades. Inappropriate utilization of these tests often leads to: (i) further investigation, (ii) physician and patient uncertainty, (iii) harm and poor outcomes, and (iv) increase in health care costs. An informed approach to the evaluation of the patients with stable ischemic chest pain can lead to efficient use of resources and better outcomes. Throughout the course of this chapter, we will explain how the applications of age-old statistical principles are still relevant in this modern era of technological advancement.

Keywords: Bayes' theorem, coronary artery disease, ischemic heart disease, appropriate use criteria

1. Introduction

Cardiovascular diseases (CVDs) remain a leading cause of death across the world [1]. Ischemic heart disease (IHD) is one of the largest contributors to these deaths both globally and in the United States of America [2] and contributes to years of productivity loss due to complications from disease sequelae. These include non-fatal myocardial infarction, stable angina pectoris and symptomatic ischemic cardiomyopathy. Although the number of deaths resulting from fatal MI has been decreasing, the number of quality years lost from IHD complications has been increasing [3]. The decrease in mortality is largely due to interventions for the management of acute coronary syndromes (ACS) and early percutaneous coronary intervention (PCI) for ST-segment elevation MI [4, 5].

There are a variety of scoring systems/tools which have been used to predict (with varying degrees of success), which patients are likely to have obstructive coronary artery disease as a cause of their chest pain [6].

The most frequently used clinical decision making tool to decide the likelihood of CAD on the basis of patient characteristics, is the Diamond-Forrester classification [7]. It is derived from the application of Bayesian principles [8] and has formed the backbone of many of the guideline statements for the management of patients with suspected stable ischemic heart disease [9, 10].

Due to the limitations of the history and physical examination in determining the likelihood of disease, clinicians have utilized various testing modalities

IntechOpen

to further increase certainty. Evaluation of chest pain has been no different. The number of available testing strategies has increased over the last few decades, and the technologies underlying these tests are constantly being refined. Despite the growing number of options, many clinicians remain unsure how to utilize these modalities [5, 11]. The increasing utilization of these tests often leads to: (i) further investigation, (ii) physician and patient uncertainty/anxiety [12], (iii) harm and (iv) increase in health care costs.

We aim to cover the following in our chapter review:

    i. Briefly simplify the principles of Bayes' theorem. Give a brief overview of the concepts of how the post-test probability of disease varies based on pre-test likelihood and test characteristics.

    ii. Review key stratification methods for the likelihood of significant CAD.

    iii. Outline the test characteristics of the main functional and anatomic imaging modalities used in chest pain evaluation based on available evidence.

    iv. Use practical examples to show how the use of low sensitivity/specificity testing in varying patient groups can lead to post-test uncertainty and the need for further testing.

    v. Explain how many of the currently available appropriate use criteria guiding testing, conflict with Bayesian principles.

Bayes' theorem has been previously applied in many clinical scenarios, including the evaluation of chest pain [13–16]. This chapter will neither be burdened with complex statistical formulas nor difficult to follow calculations. Rather, it will provide a practical approach to decision making and dealing with diagnostic uncertainty in patients with stable chest pain. Though many of the concepts expressed here are not original to the authors, we hope that this review will provide a comprehensive approach to testing—considering patient outcomes and resource utilization. The almost three century old principles of the Bayesian approach to decision making are just as relevant today with the growing technological advancements in the new era of precision medicine.

2. Bayesian approaches in clinical decision making

2.1 Clinicians and statistics

Health-care professionals at all levels of training and expertise often struggle with conceptualizing many statistical and probability ideas [17, 18]. Even for the most experienced mathematicians, the complex calculations involved in large decision making scenarios using Bayesian approaches are hard to comprehend, far less compute [13].

To follow Bayesian approaches in clinical decision making, it does require the understanding of some key statistical concepts. We hope to present this in an easy to follow format that is based in evidence [19].

The widely referenced Harvard Medical School cognitive experiment (see Appendix A) (and the research which followed) has provided much useful insight into how we approach probability testing. Two of these insights are:

i. Medical professionals often fall victim to what is referred to as the "base-rate neglect" fallacy. Here-in they place unwarranted reliability to the outcome of a test—positive or negative, ignoring the relevance of prevalence in the population.

Stated differently: A positive test result for a rare disease is more likely to be a false positive, regardless of how well the test can detect the presence of disease (sensitivity). The converse is also true, that a negative test result in a population in which there is a very high prevalence, is more likely to be a false negative.

ii. When results are presented as frequencies rather than probabilities, they are easier to follow. Take this example from Fenton and colleagues [13]:

1. Out of 1 million people 1000 are likely to die from treatment A, but only 10 are likely to die from treatment B.

Instead of:

2. The probability of dying from treatment A is 0.001, but the probability of dying from treatment B is 0.00001.

Before applying Bayes' theorem to the evaluation of chest pain, we will review some of the key statistical and probability concepts necessary to gain an understanding of Bayesian approaches.

2.2 The characteristics of diagnostic tests

There are a few characteristics of diagnostic tests which are paramount to the understanding and use of Bayesian arguments. These include sensitivity, specificity, positive predictive value, negative predictive value and likelihood ratios. There are many factors which influence the reliability or these values.

Sensitivity and specificity are often explained in complex statistical terminology, however, they can be defined very simply:

- **Sensitivity (Sens.):** The ability to pick up disease when disease is present

- **Specificity (Spec.):** The ability to rule out disease when there is no disease

Let us use the example of a hypothetical test designed to detect patients with CAD called 'CAD Finder'. We have two Groups of patients, Groups A and B (**Figure 1**). The 100 patients in Group A have proven CAD and the 100 in Group B are proven to be without CAD. To measure the sensitivity of the 'CAD Finder' we use it on patients in Group A and see how many have a positive result (93%). This is the sensitivity of the 'CAD Finder' for picking up CAD. To measure specificity, we perform the 'CAD Finder' on Group B and see how many have a negative result (80%). This would be the specificity for the 'CAD Finder' for ruling out CAD. It should also be noticed that, 7 out of 100 patients with CAD will falsely test negative and 20 out of 100 without CAD will get a false positive result.

The sensitivity and specificity of any test or maneuver are usually compared to a "gold-standard" test. In the case of suspected coronary artery disease, that test is invasive coronary angiography.

In clinical practice, it is often more helpful to gauge the performance of a test based on the prevalence of the disease of interest. This introduces the concepts of positive and negative predictive value [15].

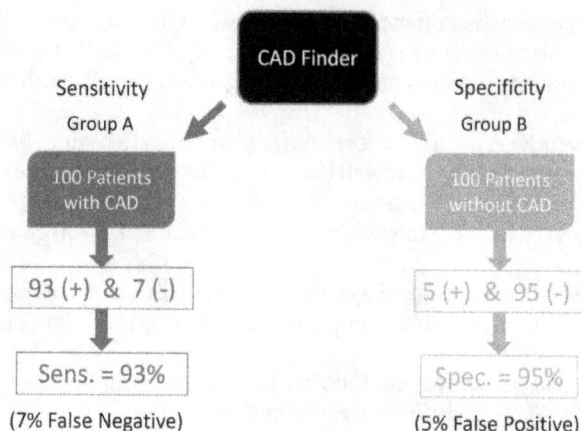

Figure 1.
Percentage of persons classified with and without CAD by the CAD finder.

- **Positive predictive value (PPV):** The ability of a test to be positive when disease truly is present.

- **Negative predictive value (NPV):** The ability of a test to be negative when disease truly is absent.

PPV and NPV vary inversely with the prevalence of a disease in a population. The relevance of this becomes apparent when tests which have been "studied" in a subgroup are applied in another population with different characteristics and disease prevalence. This brings us to our final concept worth defining:

- **Likelihood ratios:** "the likelihood that a given test result would be expected in a patient with the target disorder compared to the likelihood that that same result would be expected in a patient without the target disorder." [20]

  Using the formula:

  LR+ = sensitivity/(1-specificity).

2.3 The importance of disease prevalence, population characteristics and cut-off values

The reliability of a test is dependent on the prevalence of the disease of interest in the population in which it is studied. Bayesian methods allow us to apply known test characteristics to any population, once the population characteristics and prevalence of disease is known.

We will illustrate the outcomes when the same hypothetical test 'CAD Finder' is used in two different populations: (i) male Olympic sprinters (**Table 1**) and (ii) male elderly veterans (**Table 2**). Continuing with our hypothetical exercise, it is noted that our 'CAD Finder' is best at differentiating between 'disease' and 'no disease'.

Let us say that in a population of male Olympic sprinters, 5% have significant CAD and 95% were without. At the cut-off point for a positive result—93% of the 'Significant CAD' disease group would test positive (true positive) but 20% of the 'No CAD' group would also test positive (false positive). If the CAD Finder is used on a population of 10,000 similar Olympic sprinters, the outcomes would be as shown in **Table 1**.

Number of male Olympic sprinters with 'significant CAD' and 'No CAD' detected by the 'CAD Finder' test.					
	(93% True Positives; 20% False Positives)				
'CAD Finder' result	Actual CAD Status				Total Predicted
	Significant CAD		No CAD		
	No.	%	No.	%	
Positive	465 (TP)	93	1,900 (FP)	20	2,365
Negative	35 (FN)	7	7,600 (TN)	80	7,635
Total	500	100	9,500	100	10,000

Table 1.
Number of persons classified with 'significant CAD' and 'No CAD' by a CAD Finder Test among a population of male Olympic sprinters (low prevalence population) (93% True Positives (465); 20% False Positives (1900)).

Number of male veterans with 'significant CAD' and 'No CAD' detected by the 'CAD Finder' test.					
	(93% True Positives; 20% False Positives)				
'CAD Finder' result	Actual CAD Status				Total Predicted
	Significant CAD		No CAD		
	No.	%	No.	%	
Positive	8,835 (TP)	93	100 (FP)	20	8,935
Negative	665 (FN)	7	400 (TN)	80	1,065
Total	9,500	100	500	100	10,000

Table 2.
Number of persons classified with 'significant CAD' and 'No CAD' by a CAD finder test among a population of male veterans (high prevalence population) (80% True Negatives (400); 7% False Negatives (665)).

2.3.1 Performance of the 'CAD finder' in detecting significant CAD

When our 'CAD Finder' is used on our population of 10,000 Olympic sprinters, 2365 would test positive. However, only 465 out of those 2365 (20%) truly have significant CAD. This means that 1900 athletes will be false positives.

Rule 1. If a disease is uncommon in a population (i.e.) low prevalence—in this case 5% prevalence, any positives are more likely to be false positives.

In the population of male elderly veterans 95% have significant CAD and 5% are without disease. The outcomes of the 'CAD Finder' on a population of 10,000 similar male veterans would be depicted below in **Table 2**.

Out of the 1065 veterans who test negative for CAD, 665 (62%) actually have significant CAD. This is a large proportion of false negative results. Compare that to the population of Olympic sprinters where 35 out of the 7635 negative test results (<1%) are false negatives.

Rule 2. If a disease is highly prevalent in a population, in this case 95%, any negatives are more likely to be false negatives.

2.3.2 Performance of the 'CAD finder' in detecting persons without CAD

Since 95% of the population of athletes (9500) are truly without significant CAD, in the absence of any testing at all, if you told a patient in this population, they were without disease you would be correct most of the time. However, if we relied on our 'CAD Finder', our ability to detect athletes without CAD decreases from 95 to 76.3% (7635 of our Olympic sprinters test negative).

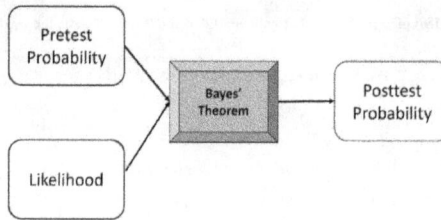

Figure 2.
Processing information using Bayes' theorem.

This illustrates that in this population of Olympic sprinters, our CAD Finder test performs very unreliably despite its good characteristics (Sensitivity 93%, Specificity 80%).

Rule 3. A test is unreliable in picking up disease when the prevalence of disease in the population is less than the value of the 'false positive rate/true positive rate'.

In our above example with the 'CAD Finder', the false positive/true positive rate = 20/93; =21%.

2.4 The Bayesian method

2.4.1 What is Bayes' theorem

Bayes' theorem (or more accurately Bayes' Rule) [21] was first described by the 18th century Episcopal minister Thomas Bayes in an essay published in the *Philosophical Transactions of the Royal Society of London* in 1764, in which he describes solving a complex problem of chances involving billiard balls [22]. Since Bayes' theorem was first theorized, it has been expressed in a variety of ways. We will use three [3] formats that are relevant to our discussion.

In mathematical terms, Bayes' theorem is expressed as follows:

$$\Pr(A|X) = \frac{\Pr(X|A)\,\Pr(A)}{\Pr(X|A)\,\Pr(A) + \Pr(X|\sim A)\,\Pr(\sim A)}$$

In this formula $\Pr(A|X)$ is the chance of having disease (A) given a positive test (X); $\Pr(X|A)$ is the chance of a positive test (X) given the presence of disease (A); $\Pr(A)$ is the pretest probability of the disease; $\Pr(\sim A)$ is the pretest probability of not having disease and $\Pr(X|\sim A)$ is the chance of a positive test (X) even if there is no disease ($\sim A$).

In plain English, Bayes' theorem states: "The probability of having a disease based on a selected test (after the test is done), is related to the pre-test probability that the patient has the disease (or its prevalence) and the test's sensitivity and specificity."

In diagrammatic form (**Figure 2**), the posttest probability is proportional to the pretest probability times the likelihood of the disease in the population. This generates the simplest representation of Bayesian statistics:

3. Practical use of Bayesian principles in cardiovascular testing

Given that accurate application of Bayes' statistics relies on the updating of probabilities (based on the acquisition of new evidence)—it is obvious then that any recommendations stated hereafter are as current as the present medical knowledge and is influenced by the writers. Our aim therefore is not to provide guidelines on the evaluation of patients with stable chest pain, but to convey a sense of comfort with using these tools, to allow the reader to generate their own informed approach to patient care.

There are generally two aims of performing cardiac testing in patients with stable chest pain (i) to determine which patients are likely to have obstructive CAD and (ii) to predict outcome or prognosis. In our discussion that follows, we will review how current testing modalities achieve either or both targets.

3.1 Determining pre-test probability in patients with stable chest pain

There are many factors which must be accounted for by the clinician when determining the pre-test probability of a patient (without known CAD) having coronary artery disease as a cause of their chest pain. These include history, patient characteristics, physical examination findings, physician experience, bias/heuristics among others. Approaches to rule-out other cardiac and non-cardiac causes will not be covered here.

We will focus on only one approach (Diamond-Forrester classification) to the generation of pre-test probability data [7], see **Tables 3** and **4**. This risk prediction model was generated through Bayesian statistics. Other scoring methods include the Goldman Reilly criteria (Goldstein), Thrombolysis in Myocardial Infarction (TIMI) risk score and the Morise Score [23]. Although it was developed over three decades ago, the Diamond-Forrester classification has been validated in modern populations [24]. The Diamond-Forrester classification stratifies patient pretest probability on the basis of three clinical variables: age, gender and chest pain characteristics. It allows clinicians to stratify patients along a spectrum of pretest likelihoods from 2 to 94%. For simplicity, many guideline groups have chosen to categorize patients in groups of very low, low, intermediate and high pretest probability (see **Table 4**). This classification of pretest probability (very low, low, intermediate and high) will form our basis of using Bayesian methods to select testing in patients.

3.2 Testing modalities for the evaluation of stable chest pain

The tests available for the evaluation of patients with stable chest pain can be divided into functional or anatomic. This is based on the type of information provided. The list of functional tests includes exercise ECG, stress echocardiogram, myocardial perfusion imaging (single-photon emission tomography (SPECT) and positron emission tomography (PET)) and stress MRI. The list of anatomic tests includes coronary CT angiography and coronary artery calcium scoring and the gold standard test-cardiac catheterization.

In **Table 5**, we have included the characteristics of the testing modalities we will reference throughout this chapter [23]. Please note that for each testing modality in **Table 5**, two values are reported for each test characteristic (sensitivity, specificity etc.)

Age, y	Nonanginal Chest Pain Men	Women	Atypical Angina Men	Women	Typical Angina Men	Women
30–39	4	2	34	12	76	26
40–49	13	3	51	22	87	55
50–59	20	7	65	31	93	73
60–69	27	14	72	51	94	86

Table 3.
Pretest likelihood of CAD in Symptomatic patients according to age and sex (combined Diamond/Forrester and CASS Data) [9].

Age (years)	Sex	Typical/Definite Angina Pectoris	Atypical/Probable Angina Pectoris	Nonanginal Chest Pain
≤39	Men	Intermediate	Intermediate	Low
	Women	Intermediate	Very low	Very low
40–49	Men	High	Intermediate	Intermediate
	Women	Intermediate	Low	Very low
50–59	Men	High	Intermediate	Intermediate
	Women	Intermediate	Intermediate	Low
≥60	Men	High	Intermediate	Intermediate
	Women	High	Intermediate	Intermediate

Table 4.
Diamond and Forrester pre-test probability of coronary artery disease by age, sex and symptoms [11].

Test	Population	Sensitivity	Specificity	PPV	NPV	LR +	LR -	Prevalence
Exercise Electrocardiography	Overall	67%	46%	41%	72%	NR	NR	NR
	Suspected CAD	62%	68%	57%	72%	1.94	0.56	41%
Stress Echocardiography	Overall	84–87%	72–77%	85–89%	69–73%	3.08–3.65	0.18–0.21	66–68%
	Suspected CAD	88%	89%	93%	80%	8.35	0.13	64%
Single Photon Emission Computed Tomography	Overall	83–85%	77–85%	79–85%	79–85%	3.56–5.13	0.18–0.22	50%
	Suspected CAD	83–84%	79–85%	72–85%	84%	3.88–5.01	0.19–0.21	41%
Positron Emission Tomography	Overall	82–90%	86–88%	93–96%	53–84%	5.57–5.88	0.11–0.21	63–80%
	Suspected CAD	90–91%	82–91%	94%	75–84%	4.97–8.89	0.11	75%
Stress Magnetic Resonance Imaging	Overall	83%	86%	94%	68%	5.93	0.20	71%
	Suspected CAD	81%	87%	93%	70%	6.39	0.21	67%
Coronary Artery Calcium Scoring	Suspected CAD	98–99%	35–40%	65–68%	93–95%	1.51	0.04	55–56%
Coronary Computed Tomography Angiography (Low radiation dose)	Suspected CAD	100%	89%	93%	99%	9.2	0.00	58%
Coronary Computed Tomography Angiography (Radiation dose not specified)	Suspected CAD	98.2%	81.6%	90.5%	99.0%	NR	NR	59.9% (28–85%)

CAD = coronary artery disease; LR + = positive likelihood ratio; LR - = negative likelihood ratio; angiography; NPV = negative predictive value; NR = not reported; PPV = positive predictive value

Table 5.
Summary of diagnostic accuracy of noninvasive tests compared with invasive coronary angiography [23].

These values are based on the test's performance when used in the overall population vs. in patients with suspected CAD. We already know from Bayesian principles that this difference is based on varying prevalence of disease in these two groups.

One important limitation of the available data is that there are no head-to-head trials comparing the test performance of many of the pharmacological or exercise testing modalities—using cardiac catheterization as a reference. Current data is limited to small samples sizes and the use of old techniques/technologies.

3.3 Noninvasive functional tests

It is important to make the distinction between exercise testing and 'stress testing' which are often used synonymously. 'Stress testing' refers to any pharmacological or exercise testing modality which imposes a stress on the cardiovascular system [25]. Many of these alternative forms of 'stress testing' modalities will be covered in the following subsections.

3.3.1 Exercise ECG

Exercise ECG testing is often the first used testing modality in the workup of stable chest pain [11]. It has been around for several decades and has been studied in many clinical scenarios. Unfortunately, it has an intermediate sensitivity and specificity for the detection of CAD. Exercise testing is based on the premise of monitoring the cardiovascular system's response to physiological stress. This is to determine clinical signs and symptoms which would not be present at rest.

Exercise testing in the lab uses dynamic testing principles because (i) it can be graduated and (ii) it places a volume stress on the heart [25].

There are various exercise protocols available for laboratory exercise testing. The Bruce Protocol is most commonly used [26]. Regardless of the protocol, exercise capacity is graduated and measured at various "stages". This is based on the physiological principle that at a given intensity of activity, the parameters of heart rate, blood pressure, and cardiac output are relatively constant [27]. The quantity of oxygen transported and utilized in cellular metabolism is measured as VO_{2max}, which will be discussed in more detail later [28]. A second measurement parameter of oxygen utilization is myocardial oxygen uptake or Mo_2. In clinical scenarios Mo_2 is estimated by the product of heart rate and systolic blood pressure (rate-pressure product). In healthy myocardium, there is a linear relationship between Mo_2 and coronary vessel blood flow [25].

However, if there is either an obstruction to flow or reduction in myocardial cell uptake of oxygen (as in ischemia), then the Mo_2 in the region will be reduced. The implications of this are that if there is a coronary obstruction, a point will be reached where there is supply/demand mismatch and signs and symptoms of ischemia will occur. Regardless of the form of physical activity, for any given coronary obstruction, angina usually occurs at the same rate-pressure product.

The rate of oxygen uptake by healthy tissue will increase with increasing demand until it reaches a maximal level of oxygen extraction. This is termed the VO_{2max}, and varies with age (and to a lesser degree with gender). It has been observed that increasing VO_2 during exercise has a linear relationship with heart rate until it reaches the VO_{2max} plateau. At this point, the heart rate may continue to increase as myocardial energy generation reverts to anaerobic metabolism. This, in turn, may cause signs and symptoms of ischemia, which in turn may cause a 'false positive' finding for ischemia.

Most labs use the formula, 220-Age (for either gender) to calculate a Maximal Predicted Heart Rate (MPHR) as a surrogate for VO_{2max}. Target heart rates for exercise testing are then usually set at 85–100% of MPHR. In the absence of symptoms, ECG changes (or any other reasons to stop the test early), the test is routinely stopped when the MPHR is achieved. It is therefore important to recognize that exercise stress tests can have a false-negative if the level of exercise does not reach the target but may become false-positive if it reaches above the maximum.

In general, the two common exercise methods used are either the treadmill or cycle ergometer. End points for exercise include: achievement of target heart rate, fatigue, symptoms (such as chest pain or dyspnea), significant ECG changes (such as ST segment depressions or elevations), significant dysrhythmias, drop of systolic blood pressure (usually >10 mmHg), patient request or inability to continue.

The diagnosis of ischemia is usually made from chest pains and/or development of horizontal or down-sloping ST segment deviations of ≥1 mm during exercise or the recovery period. Other ECG criteria, such as the development of a bundle branch block (especially LBBB) may suggest ischemia (but are less sensitive).

In addition to evaluation for ischemia, the exertional capacity and hemodynamic responses to stress testing have additional prognostic value [26]. One of the more popular ways to evaluate this is with the Duke Treadmill Score (DTS), which incorporates exertional capacity, ECG changes and symptom onset (*Exercise minutes (Bruce)* − (*ST deviation in mm X 5*) − (*angina index X 4*)) [29].

There are several limitations to standard exercise stress testing. Firstly, it is limited by a patient's ability to exercise and achieve the target heart rate. Additionally, any baseline ECG abnormalities, such as left bundle branch block, left ventricular hypertrophy with repolarization abnormalities, ST segment depression and ventricular pre-excitation, further reduces the test's specificity and even sensitivity [26].

The use of image testing as an adjunct to exercise testing, improves both sensitivity and specificity. Imaging with the use of pharmacologic agents can also be useful in patients who cannot ambulate or have baseline ECG abnormalities limiting interpretation. Currently, the most commonly used stress imaging modalities are echocardiography and nuclear imaging.

3.3.2 Stress echocardiography

Stress echocardiography (SE) is reliant on the identification of wall motion and wall thickening abnormalities. Generally, patients undergo echo acquisitions prior to exercise and immediately after exercise (or, in patients who exercise on supine bicycles, at peak exercise). The images are compared between rest and stress for changes in wall motion, wall thickening and left ventricular sized and function. Sensitivities for SE are about 88%, with a specificity of 89%.

The major advantages of SE are availability, absence of radiation exposure and cost. However, it has been reported to have lower sensitivity than radionuclide imaging, especially in single vessel disease detection [30]. It is also operator dependent and image quality is limited by patient characteristics (e.g. COPD and obesity). When used with exercise testing, it is limited by the patient's ability to get into position for scanning quickly after peak exercise (typically, the patient must get off the treadmill, get in the correct position on the bed and the sonographer must acquire good images in four different views—all within 1 min).

For patients who cannot walk, dobutamine stress echocardiography (DSE) has been shown to offer similar sensitivity and specificity to SE for the detection of obstructive CAD. However, because it does not involve exercise, the additional prognostic data offered by exercise protocols (e.g. using the Duke Treadmill Score) are not available with DSE.

3.3.3 Nuclear imaging testing

There are two forms of radionuclide imaging modalities currently available for chest pain evaluation: single-photon emission tomography (SPECT) and positron emission tomography (PET). Both rely on the use of radiotracer isotopes to detect areas of ischemia or infarct. There are two types of SPECT radiotracers commonly used in clinical settings: technetium (Tc-99m)-labeled tracers and thallium (Tl-201). PET imaging uses the more high-energy rubidium (Rb)-82 radiotracer. The physical and physiological principles behind how radiotracers elements are used to evaluate for CAD is beyond the scope of this chapter. We will focus on the performance characteristics of both nuclear tests and a few pertinent advantages and disadvantages.

3.3.3.1 SPECT

SPECT imaging can be used in conjunction with exercise or pharmacologic agents to assess for CAD. When SPECT is used with exercise protocols, it provides similar functional capacity and ECG data as exercise ECG, with the added sensitivity and specificity provided by imaging. It is the more commonly used and more readily available of the radionuclide modalities.

Pharmacologic stress images are most commonly obtained with vasodilating agents (adenosine, dipyridamole and regadenoson). The vasodilating agents either differently or indirectly stimulate the A_{2A} (adenosine) receptors leading to coronary arteriolar vasodilation. Vasodilating agents are suitable for use in patients who cannot exercise, where significant increases in heart rate are not desired (e.g. patients with permanent pacemaker devices or left bundle branch block) or patients who have had recent acute coronary syndromes. Sensitivity and specificities for these are between 83–84% and 79–85% respectively.

SPECT is a great alternative to stress echocardiography, when patient's characteristics prevent good imaging windows [30, 31]. It has a number of important limitations. Since it is dependent on radiotracer delivery to tissue, in patients with equally compromised flow in all coronary vessels (triple vessel disease), there is risk for a false negative study—due to so-called 'balanced ischemia'. Soft tissue and uptake by other organs (e.g.) gallbladder can also limit image quality and often cause false positive findings [23].

3.3.3.2 PET

PET imaging uses the more high-energy rubidium (Rb)-82 radiotracer. This allows for less displacement by soft tissue and potentially fewer false positives. PET has the additional advantage of being combined with CT imaging. This allows for soft-tissue attenuation correction (to reduce false positives) and assessment of coronary artery calcium (which will be discussed later).

The major disadvantage of PET is the shorter half-life of radiotracer and its cost. As a result, its availability is limited.

3.4 Noninvasive anatomic tests

3.4.1 Coronary CT angiography (CCTA)

Coronary CT angiography allows for non-invasive assessment of coronary artery disease [32]. Intravenous contrast agents within the lumen of coronary vessels facilitate visual calculation of obstruction/stenosis. Newer CT techniques use a 64-multislide (or better) acquisition hardware to obtain images. Available post-processing software packages further refine images.

The definition of 'significant coronary artery disease' (CAD) with CT coronary angiography is $\geq$70% diameter stenosis of at least one major epicardial artery segment or $\geq$50% diameter stenosis in the left main coronary artery [33]. The presence of collateral coronary supply as well as low at-risk myocardium can render high degree stenotic lesions asymptomatic. For this reason, the degree of CAD obstruction correlates poorly with symptoms and limits its usefulness for determining the cause of chest pain.

The presence of coronary calcium causes artifacts during imaging that may obscure the coronary lumen. For this reason, CCTA is often combined with assessment of coronary calcium to make predictions about outcomes or prognosis [34]. Novel techniques such as fractional flow reserve derived from CT (FFR_{CT}) are being used to determine whether stenotic lesions are physiologically significant [35]. FFR_{CT} is beyond the scope of discussion here.

Although CCTA allows for rapid imagining, it has limited utility in patients with rapid heart rates, arrhythmias, renal impairment. It also carries radiation exposure risk.

3.4.2 Coronary artery calcium scoring (CACS)

CACS is obtained using non-contrast CT scanning. Post-processing algorithms are used to quantify the degree of coronary vessel calcification. The three most common scoring methods are Agatston, volume and mass. CAC scoring has been in formal use since 1990 [36]. Although traditionally it has been recommended for use in asymptomatic patients, it has been shown to provide similar predictive reliability as functional testing, especially when used with other CT modalities [37].

Evidence suggests that a positive CAC is more sensitive than functional testing at predicting MACE. Alternatively, an abnormal functional test result is more specific. Increasing the cut-off point of a 'positive' CAC improves specificity at the expense of sensitivity [38]. This is a consequence of the Bayesian principles we discussed. However, it has little usefulness in determining the cause of chest pain.

3.5 Bayesian approach to test selection

Using the Diamond-Forrester classification, there are three broad categories of patients with stable chest pain that a clinician will likely encounter. These are grouped as 'low pretest probability—5%', 'intermediate pre-test probability— approx. 50%' and 'high pre-test probability—95%'. In the following three subsections we will explore strategies of using Bayesian approaches to testing in each of these groups.

There are many factors which will influence real life decisions on which tests to order and when. Some of these are patient characteristics (ability to exercise), resource availability, institutional culture, and the degree of uncertainty a clinician/ patient is comfortable with accepting.

Bayesian approaches allow us to make informed decisions on sequential test selection. Tests assessing CAD by the same markers should not be duplicated. To avoid this, one potential way of classifying testing modalities would be: (i) tests that identify ischemia via surface changes—(e.g. stress ECG), (ii) tests that identify ischemia via nuclear tracer, (iii) tests that identify ischemia via wall motion abnormalities—(e.g. stress echocardiography) [15].

3.5.1 Test selection in patients with low and high pre-test probability

We know from 'Rule 1' that in a population with low prevalence, any positive result is likely to be a false positive. This means that in this scenario (low pretest probability) if one opts not to perform any cardiac testing, because you suspect the patient does not have CAD, you would be correct most of the time. 'Rule 3' stated that "If a disease is highly prevalent in a population, any negatives are more likely to be false negatives". We also learnt in Section 2 that when testing is performed in this group, the possibility of true positive results does not improve much on no testing at all. If one opted to assume that every patient in this group (high pretest probability) had significant CAD and went ahead with a definitive test/treatment (i.e. ICA), one would be correct most of the time, and may avoid an unnecessary interim test.

3.5.2 Test selection in patients with intermediate pre-test probability

The intermediate pre-test probability group is where Bayesian approaches yield the greatest benefit. This is also where informed sequential testing can be very informative and efficient if used correctly. It is impossible for us to illustrate the relative outcomes of all possible combinations of testing here. We will use two examples to illustrate how tests with varying sensitivities and specificities can give different post-test probabilities when used in high (Patient A), low (Patient B) or intermediate pre-test probability patients (Patient C).

Patient **A** has very high pre-test probability of disease (95%).
Patient **B** has very low pre-test probability of disease (5%).
Patient **C** has an intermediate probability of disease (50%).

Example 1. A test has a sensitivity of 90% and specificity 90% (e.g. nuclear imaging testing).

- Patient **A** (with 95% pre-test probability):

    ○ Chance a + test will mean + disease= >99%

    ○ Chance a − test will mean + disease = 68%

- Patient **B** (with 5% pre-test probability):

    ○ Chance a + test will mean + disease = 32%

    ○ Chance a − test will mean + disease = <1%

- Patient **C** (with 50% pre-test probability):

    ○ Chance a + test will mean + disease = 90%

    ○ Chance a − test will mean + disease = 10%

Example 2. A test has a sensitivity of 65% and specificity 65% (e.g. Exercise ECG testing).

- Patient **A** (95% pre-test probability):

    ○ Chance a + test will mean + disease = 97%

    ○ Chance a − test will mean + disease = 91%

- Patient **B** (5% pre-test probability):

    ○ Chance a + test will mean + disease = 9%

    ○ Chance a − test will mean + disease = 3%

- Patient **C** (50% pre-test probability):

    ○ Chance a + test will mean + disease = 65%

    ○ Chance a − test will mean + disease = 35%

The decision on when to stop testing or proceed with further evaluation based on post-test certainty, is highly individualized. It is based on the post-test value at which one thinks a disease has been either sufficiently 'ruled-in' or 'ruled-out'. Generally, most a pre-test or post-test probability of ≤15% or ≥85% would be considered reasons to stop further testing—and either assume no disease when the probability is ≤15% or assume disease when the probability is ≥85%.

4. Appropriate use criteria and the delivery of high-value care

Technological advancement has resulted in a growing number of available testing modalities that offer increased sensitivity and specificity [39]. This rapid growth has led to an increase in healthcare expenditure. Payers were the first to respond to this growth by implementing restrictions to regulate expenditure through strict criteria for reimbursement and prior authorization requirement.

In response, clinician led groups developed Appropriate Use Criteria (AUC) to improve efficient utilization of these testing modalities [40]. The American College of Cardiology (ACC) along with other organizations have developed AUC documents to aide with decision making for cardiac testing. The first statement of this kind was for the efficient utilization of myocardial perfusion imaging in 2005 [41]. Subsequently, AUC documents have classified indications for the use of: CCTA, echocardiography (including stress), cardiac magnetic resonance among others.

AUC documents are distinct from clinical guideline/recommendation statements. Appropriate use is classified based on the ratio of possible benefit versus the potential harm of a procedure with an eye to 'cost-effectiveness'. The definition of "an appropriate diagnostic or therapeutic procedure is one in which the expected clinical benefit exceeds the risks of the procedure by a sufficiently wide margin, such that the procedure is generally considered acceptable or reasonable care" [40].

AUC are scored from 1 to 9 and classified into three broad categories: 'rarely appropriate care' (score 1–3), 'may be appropriate care' (score 4–6) and 'appropriate care' (score 7–9). The Bayesian criticism of these AUC statements is that they are often not based on evidence but rather on aims to reduce healthcare expenditure based on the availability of less costly, safe alternatives.

5. Review of the current recommendations for the evaluation of stable ischemic heart disease (SIHD)

The use of functional testing (both exercise and pharmacological) has long been favored as the preferred modality of ischemia evaluation [10]. The main reasons are: (i) that applying increasing workload on the heart more closely mimics the pathophysiology of supply/demand mismatch, (ii) exercise capacity provides incremental diagnostic and prognostic information and finally, and (iii) cost-effectiveness.

Since the advent of exercise stress testing, many alternative diagnostic modalities have become available. As was previously mentioned, most of these testing modalities have not been compared to each other in head-to-head trials. The Bayesian criticism of much of the available evidence is that limited data regarding pretest clinical stratification or how posttest classification contributed to decision making is reported [42].

The biggest questions of the last decade have been whether (i) bypassing testing is a viable/safe option in select low risk patient groups, and (ii) if anatomic testing is as good as or a better alternative to traditional functional testing [37, 43]. It would be counterproductive to review all the guideline recommendations and AUC here since they are frequently revised and there are many competing agencies that produce them. Instead, we will just highlight a few which either follow or contradict the Bayesian method to give the reader a better understanding of some of their limitations.

In patients with low pretest probability and at low risk it is reasonable to exclude the diagnosis of stable angina on clinical assessment alone and defer further diagnostic testing [33]. This is supported by Bayesian argument. The decision to defer testing is highly individual and will be guided by physician experience and shared decision making with patients.

The AUCs recommend exercise ECG as the initial testing modality in most patient populations [9–11]. We have previously showed the potential pitfalls of low sensitivity and specificity testing in either low or high probability patients. For this reason we do not recommend that exercise ECG testing be used alone to either exclude or diagnose significant CAD as a cause of stable chest pain, no matter the pretest probability [33]. However, exercise testing is still recommended because of the valuable prognostic information it provides (with the use of Duke Treadmill Score, etc.). This leads to the other bit of contradictory recommendations in the area of stress echocardiography in low pretest groups—where a patient's ability to exercise downgrades stress echocardiography testing from 'appropriate' to 'inappropriate' [44]. Presumably, the AUC feels that a regular ECG exercise test is preferable in these patients, contrary to Bayesian arguments.

When the pretest probability of disease is very high, any testing is likely to result in a false negative. Bayesian methods argue for proceeding with definitive testing/ intervention. However, even in this patient population invasive coronary angiography is usually a second or third-line option after other non-invasive tests are inconclusive [9, 33].

The anatomic testing modalities have high sensitivity. Nevertheless, they are regarded as rarely appropriate across all patient groups by current AUC [11]. On the other hand, the current NICE guidelines recommend offering 64-slice CCTA as a first testing modality in patients with typical angina. The recommendations for Heartflow FFR_{CT} are less clear [45].

The final question remains, what is regarded as 'confirmatory'. This varies with clinician comfort and experience. Some guidelines suggest that a posttest probability of >85% is sufficient to confirm the diagnosis of significant CAD [15].

6. Limitations of the Bayesian approach

One of the major limitations of the use of the Bayesian method is its reliance on pre-test probability (some advocates of Bayesian approaches consider this to be a strength). Many critics have stated that this results in 'subjectivity' on which inferences of post-test outcomes are based [42]. We have already stated some of the many factors which contribute to variations in pre-test estimates at the individual clinician level. This point just reiterates the importance of scrutinizing the quality of evidence on which conclusions are based. Other proponents of the Bayesian approach have therefore stressed the need to base pre-test probability on sound reasoning and evidence and to combine available data to reach consensus [42].

7. Conclusions

Bayesian analysis is very important in the evaluation of patients with stable ischemic chest pain. Even with the use of a simplified assessment tool of pretest probabilities, one can maximize efficiency of test selection, lower costs and improve patient outcomes.

Conflict of interest

The authors have no conflicts of interest to declare.

Appendices and Nomenclature

"One in thousand people have a prevalence for a particular heart disease. There is a test to detect this disease. The test is 100% accurate for people who have the disease, and is 95% accurate for those who do not (this means that 5% of people who do not have the disease will be wrongly diagnosed as having it). If a randomly selected person tests positive what is the probability that the person actually has the disease?"

Author details

John-Ross D. Clarke[1*] and Gilead I. Lancaster[2,3]

1 Department of Internal Medicine, Yale-New Haven Health - Bridgeport Hospital, Bridgeport, CT, USA

2 Heart and Vascular Center, Yale-New Haven Health - Bridgeport Hospital, Bridgeport, CT, USA

3 Yale University School of Medicine, New Haven, CT, USA

*Address all correspondence to: johnrossclarke@gmail.com

IntechOpen

References

[1] Roth GA, Johnson C, Abajobir A, Abd-Allah F, Abera SF, Abyu G, et al. Global, regional, and national burden of cardiovascular diseases for 10 causes, 1990 to 2015. Journal of the American College of Cardiology. 2017;**70**(1):1-25

[2] Mathers CD, Loncar D. Projections of global mortality and burden of disease from 2002 to 2030. PLoS Medicine. 2006;**3**(11):e442

[3] Moran AE, Forouzanfar MH, Roth GA, Mensah GA, Ezzati M, Flaxman A, et al. The global burden of ischemic heart disease in 1990 and 2010: The global burden of disease 2010 study. Circulation. 2014;**129**(14):1493-1501

[4] Amsterdam EA, Wenger NK, Brindis RG, Casey DE Jr, Ganiats TG, Holmes DR Jr, et al. AHA/ACC Guideline for the management of patients with non-ST-elevation acute coronary syndromes: A report of the American College of Cardiology/American Heart Association Task Force on Practice Guidelines. Journal of the American College of Cardiology. 2014, 2014;**64**(24):e139-e228

[5] Coronary Revascularization Writing Group, Patel MR, Dehmer GJ, Hirshfeld JW, Smith PK, Spertus JA, et al. ACCF/SCAI/STS/AATS/AHA/ASNC/HFSA/SCCT 2012 appropriate use criteria for coronary revascularization focused update: A report of the American College of Cardiology Foundation Appropriate Use Criteria Task Force, Society for Cardiovascular Angiography and Interventions, Society of Thoracic Surgeons, American Association for Thoracic Surgery, American Heart Association, American Society of Nuclear Cardiology, and the Society of Cardiovascular Computed Tomography. The Journal of Thoracic and Cardiovascular Surgery. 2012;**143**(4):780-803

[6] Hamburger RF, Spertus JA, Winchester DE. Utility of the Diamond-Forrester classification in stratifying acute chest pain in an academic chest pain center. Critical Pathways in Cardiology. 2016;**15**(2):56-59

[7] Diamond GA, Forrester JS. Analysis of probability as an aid in the clinical diagnosis of coronary-artery disease. The New England Journal of Medicine. 1979;**300**(24):1350-1358

[8] Graham IM. Diagnosing coronary artery disease: The Diamond and Forrester model revisited. European Heart Journal. 2011;**32**(11):1311-1312

[9] Fihn SD, Blankenship JC, Alexander KP, Bittl JA, Byrne JG, Fletcher BJ, et al. ACC/AHA/AATS/PCNA/SCAI/STS focused update of the guideline for the diagnosis and management of patients with stable ischemic heart disease: A report of the American College of Cardiology/American Heart Association Task Force on Practice Guidelines, and the American Association for Thoracic Surgery, Preventive Cardiovascular Nurses Association, Society for Cardiovascular Angiography and Interventions, and Society of Thoracic Surgeons. Circulation. 2014, 2014;**130**(19):1749-1767

[10] Fihn SD, Gardin JM, Abrams J, Berra K, Blankenship JC, Dallas AP, et al. ACCF/AHA/ACP/AATS/PCNA/SCAI/STS guideline for the diagnosis and management of patients with stable ischemic heart disease: A report of the American College of Cardiology Foundation/American Heart Association task force on practice guidelines, and the American College of Physicians, American Association for Thoracic Surgery, Preventive Cardiovascular Nurses Association, Society for Cardiovascular Angiography and Interventions, and Society of

Thoracic Surgeons. Circulation. 2012, 2012;**126**(25):e354-e471

[11] Wolk MJ, Bailey SR, Doherty JU, Douglas PS, Hendel RC, Kramer CM, et al. ACCF/AHA/ASE/ASNC/HFSA/HRS/SCAI/SCCT/SCMR/STS 2013 multimodality appropriate use criteria for the detection and risk assessment of stable ischemic heart disease: A report of the American College of Cardiology Foundation Appropriate Use Criteria Task Force, American Heart Association, American Society of Echocardiography, American Society of Nuclear Cardiology, Heart Failure Society of America, Heart Rhythm Society, Society for Cardiovascular Angiography and Interventions, Society of Cardiovascular Computed Tomography, Society for Cardiovascular Magnetic Resonance, and Society of Thoracic Surgeons. Journal of the American College of Cardiology. 2014;**63**(4):380-406

[12] Gigerenzer G. Reckoning with Risk: Learning to Live with Uncertainty. United Kingdom: Penguin Books Limited; 2003

[13] Fenton N, Neil M. Comparing risks of alternative medical diagnosis using Bayesian arguments. Journal of Biomedical Informatics. 2010;**43**(4):485-495

[14] Col NF, Ngo L, Fortin JM, Goldberg RJ, O'Connor AM. Can computerized decision support help patients make complex treatment decisions? A randomized controlled trial of an individualized menopause decision aid. Medical Decision Making. 2007;**27**(5):585-598

[15] Owen A. Bayes theorem and diagnostic tests with application to patients with suspected angina. International Cardiovascular Forum Journal. 2015;**1**(2):96-100

[16] Detrano R, Yiannikas J, Salcedo EE, Rincon G, Go RT, Williams G, et al. Bayesian probability analysis: A prospective demonstration of its clinical utility in diagnosing coronary disease. Circulation. 1984;**69**(3):541-547

[17] Casscells W, Schoenberger A, Graboys TB. Interpretation by physicians of clinical laboratory results. The New England Journal of Medicine. 1978;**299**(18):999-1001

[18] Eddy DM, Kahneman D, Slovic P, Tversky A. Probabilistic reasoning in clinical medicine: Problems and opportunities. In: Judgment under uncertainty. United Kingdom: Cambridge University Press; 1982. pp. 249-267

[19] Cosmides L. Are humans good intuitive statisticians after all? Rethinking some conclusions from the literature on judgment under uncertainty. Cognition. 1996;**58**(1):1-73

[20] CEBM. Likelihood Ratios. 2014. Available from: https://www.cebm.net/2014/02/likelihood-ratios/

[21] Hacking I. An Introduction to Probability and Inductive Logic. United Kingdom: Cambridge University Press; 2001

[22] Westbury CF. Bayes' rule for clinicians: An introduction. Frontiers in Psychology. 2010;**1**:192

[23] Skelly AC, Hashimoto R, Buckley DI, Brodt ED, Noelck N, Totten AM, et al. Noninvasive Testing for Coronary Artery Disease. Comparative Effectiveness Review No. 171. 2016. Available from: www.effectivehealthcare.ahrq.gov/reports/final.cfm

[24] Genders TS, Steyerberg EW, Hunink MG, Nieman K, Galema TW, Mollet NR, et al. Prediction model to estimate presence of coronary artery disease: Retrospective pooled analysis of existing cohorts. BMJ. 2012;**344**:e3485

[25] Fletcher GF, Balady G, Froelicher VF, Hartley LH, Haskell WL, Pollock ML. Exercise standards. A statement for healthcare professionals from the American Heart Association Writing Group. Circulation. 1995;**91**(2):580-615

[26] Gibbons RJ, Balady GJ, Timothy Bricker J, Chaitman BR, Fletcher GF, Froelicher VF, et al. ACC/AHA 2002 guideline update for exercise testing: Summary article. Journal of the American College of Cardiology. 2002;**40**(8):1531-1540

[27] Nixon PGF. Human circulation regulation during physical stress. L. B. Rowell. Oxford University Press, London, 1986. No. of pages: 416. Price: £35.00. Stress Medicine. 1988;**4**(2):124-125

[28] Myers J, Madhavan R. Exercise testing with gas exchange analysis. Cardiology Clinics. 2001;**19**(3):433-445

[29] Mark DB, Hlatky MA, Harrell FE Jr, Lee KL, Califf RM, Pryor DB. Exercise treadmill score for predicting prognosis in coronary artery disease. Annals of Internal Medicine. 1987;**106**(6):793-800

[30] Fleischmann KE, Hunink MGM, Kuntz KM, Douglas PS. Exercise echocardiography or exercise SPECT imaging? Journal of the American Medical Association. 1998;**280**(10):913-920

[31] Kim C, Kwok YS, Heagerty P, Redberg R. Pharmacologic stress testing for coronary disease diagnosis: A meta-analysis. American Heart Journal. 2001;**142**(6):934-944

[32] Arbab-Zadeh A, Miller JM, Rochitte CE, Dewey M, Niinuma H, Gottlieb I, et al. Diagnostic accuracy of computed tomography coronary angiography according to pre-test probability of coronary artery disease and severity of coronary arterial calcification. The CORE-64 (Coronary artery evaluation using 64-row multidetector computed tomography angiography) International Multicenter Study. Journal of the American College of Cardiology. 2012;**59**(4):379-387

[33] NICE. Chest Pain of Recent Onset: Assessment and Diagnosis, 2010 July 2. 2019. Available from: www.nice.org.uk/guidance/cg95

[34] Abbara S, Arbab-Zadeh A, Callister TQ, Desai MY, Mamuya W, Thomson L, et al. SCCT guidelines for performance of coronary computed tomographic angiography: A report of the Society of Cardiovascular Computed Tomography Guidelines Committee. Journal of Cardiovascular Computed Tomography. 2009;**3**(3):190-204

[35] Asher A, Singhal A, Thornton G, Wragg A, Davies C. FFRCT derived from computed tomography angiography: The experience in the UK. Expert Review of Cardiovascular Therapy. 2018;**16**(12):919-929

[36] Blaha MJ, Mortensen MB, Kianoush S, Tota-Maharaj R, Cainzos-Achirica M. Coronary artery calcium scoring: Is it time for a change in methodology? JACC: Cardiovascular Imaging. 2017;**10**(8):923-937

[37] Douglas PS, Hoffmann U, Patel MR, Mark DB, Al-Khalidi HR, Cavanaugh B, et al. Outcomes of anatomical versus functional testing for coronary artery disease. The New England Journal of Medicine. 2015;**372**(14):1291-1300

[38] Hoffmann U, Ferencik M, Udelson JE, Picard MH, Truong QA, Patel MR, et al. Prognostic value of noninvasive cardiovascular testing in patients with stable chest pain: Insights from the PROMISE trial (prospective multicenter imaging study for evaluation of chest pain). Circulation. 2017;**135**(24):2320-2332

[39] Iglehart JK. Health insurers and medical-imaging policy--a work in progress. The New England Journal of Medicine. 2009;**360**(10):1030-1037

[40] Hendel RC, Lindsay BD, Allen JM, Brindis RG, Patel MR, White L, et al. ACC appropriate use criteria methodology: 2018 update: A report of the American College of Cardiology Appropriate Use Criteria Task Force. Journal of the American College of Cardiology. 2018;**71**(8):935-948

[41] Brindis RG, Douglas PS, Hendel RC, Peterson ED, Wolk MJ, Allen JM, et al. ACCF/ASNC appropriateness criteria for single-photon emission computed tomography myocardial perfusion imaging (SPECT MPI): A report of the American College of Cardiology Foundation Quality Strategic Directions Committee Appropriateness Criteria Working Group and the American Society of Nuclear Cardiology endorsed by the American Heart Association. Journal of the American College of Cardiology. 2005;**46**(8):1587-1605

[42] O'Hagan A. Bayesian Statistics: Principles and Benefits. Dordrecht: Springer; 2004. pp. 31-45

[43] Investigators S-H, Newby DE, Adamson PD, Berry C, Boon NA, Dweck MR, et al. Coronary CT angiography and 5-year risk of myocardial infarction. The New England Journal of Medicine. 2018;**379**(10):924-933

[44] American College of Cardiology Foundation Appropriate Use Criteria Task Force, American Society of Echocardiography, American Heart Association, American Society of Nuclear Cardiology, Heart Failure Society of America, Heart Rhythm Society, et al. ACCF/ASE/AHA/ASNC/ HFSA/HRS/SCAI/SCCM/SCCT/ SCMR 2011 Appropriate Use Criteria for Echocardiography. A report of the American College of Cardiology Foundation Appropriate Use Criteria Task Force, American Society of Echocardiography, American Heart Association, American Society of Nuclear Cardiology, Heart Failure Society of America, Heart Rhythm Society, Society for Cardiovascular Angiography and Interventions, Society of Critical Care Medicine, Society of Cardiovascular Computed Tomography, Society for Cardiovascular Magnetic Resonance American College of Chest Physicians. Journal of the American Society of Echocardiography. 2011;**24**(3):229-267

[45] NICE. HeartFlow FFRCT for Estimating Fractional Flow Reserve From Coronary CT Angiography, 2017 July 2. 2019. Available from: nice.org.uk/ guidance/mtg32

Approach to Gastroesophageal Reflux: A Cause of Chest Pain in Infants with Congenital Heart Disease

Mehmet Semih Demirtaş

Abstract

The life expectancy and quality of life of infants with congenital heart disease have increased in the last 30 years with significant advances in technological facilities, treatment methods, and surgeries. GER is a condition that can be seen in infants with CHD, which needs to be well followed up and to be differentiated between physiological and nonphysiological reflux. GER is a physiological condition that is common in infants with CHD and usually resolves spontaneously in the first 6–12 months of life. If the baby has adequate weight gain and nutrition status and there is no abnormal restlessness, the baby is considered to be uncomplicated GER. GERD is a pathological clinical entity that is accompanied by insufficient weight gain, esophagitis, and persistent respiratory system findings. When gastroesophageal reflux disease is considered, the first thing to be done is to complete the detailed anamnesis and physical examination of the infant. The reflux status of the infants can be examined with the surveys that were prepared for GERD and followed up for 1–2 months. If necessary, diagnostic methods such as esophageal pH monitoring and radiological and endoscopic examinations can be used. Conservative approaches such as thickening of formulas and thickening of formulas and positional feeding are the the first treatment approaches for reflux.

Keywords: congenital heart disease, gastroesophageal reflux disease, infant, treatment, surveys

1. Introduction

The prevalence of congenital heart disease (CHD) is known to be approximately 0.5–0.8% in all live births [1]. It is estimated that approximately 30–35% of children with CHD require medical treatment, interventional procedures, or surgical treatment [2]. Over the last 30 years, significant advances in surgical techniques and medical treatment have been made in the treatment of CHD in the world [3]. Nutritional status of CHD patients in the first year has an important role in growth and neurodevelopmental functions. GERD, which is closely related to nutrition and malnutrition, should be considered in these patients [4].

Gastroesophageal reflux is a common condition in children in all age groups, with gastric contents retrograde passage to the esophagus, even pharynx and mouth. This condition is defined as gastroesophageal reflux disease (GERD) if it continues more frequently and continuously and causes worrisome symptoms and undesirable consequences [5]. Especially, it results in esophagitis or other esophageal symptoms or symptoms of the respiratory system.

2. Definition

Gastroesophageal reflux is a physiological condition that may occur in healthy infants, children, and adults. It usually occurs in very short episodes (<3 minutes) and in the postprandial period without any symptom, esophageal damage, or complications. If these reflux processes cause worrisome symptoms and unwanted conditions, GERD is in question [6, 7].

Regurgitation refers to reflux in the oropharynx, while vomiting refers to the gastric contents coming out of the mouth. There is no need to be with repetition and any coercion. The use of these terms is intertwined in clinical practice, and no definite distinction is made. They are perceived as different states of the same process. Symptoms occur for many reasons (**Table 1**).

Causes of vomiting		
Gastrointestinal obstruction	**Neurological**	**Renal**
Pyloric stenosis	Hydrocephalus	Obstructive uropathy
Malrotation	Subdural hematoma	Renal insufficiency
Intestinal duplication	Intracranial hemorrhage	
Hirschsprung's disease	Intracranial mass	**Toxic**
Antral/duodenal web	Infant migraine	The lead
Foreign body	Chiari malformation	Iron
		Vitamins A and D
Other gastrointestinal causes	**Infectious**	**Cardiac**
Achalasia	Sepsis	Congestive heart failure
Gastroparesis	Meningitis	Vascular ring
Gastroenteritis	Urinary infection	
Peptic ulcer	Pneumonia	**Metabolic/endocrine**
Eosinophilic esophagitis	Otitis media	Galactosemia
gastroenteritis		Hereditary fructose intolerance
Food allergy		Urea cycle defects
		Amino and organic acidemias
		Congenital adrenal hyperplasia

Table 1.
Differential diagnosis in vomiting infants.

3. Epidemiology

A study of 948 infants in the United States reported a prevalence of reflux in the 4–6 months of life as 67% which has decreased to 5% by 10–12 months of age. Similarly in the study with 602 babies in India, it showed that the prevalence of gastroesophageal reflux, which was 55% in the first 6 months of life, decreased to 4% at 1 year of age [8, 9]. Epidemiological studies suggest that gastroesophageal reflux in infancy with CHD can be seen from the first month of life and the frequency of occurrence reaches to the peak around the fourth month, most of them recover after the age of 1 year, almost all of them at the age of 2 [10].

There is also a genetic predisposition to GERD. In addition to known GERD symptoms in some families, the incidence of endoscopic esophagitis, hiatus hernia, Barrett's esophagus, and adenocarcinoma has been shown [11, 12]. Genetic factors which the 9q22-9q31 gene was mapped with infantile gastroesophageal reflux were thought to play a role in the concordance of gastroesophageal reflux in monozygotic twins compared to dizygotic twins [13].

Regurgitation is common in infants. However, typically around 1 year of age, it decreases or completely recovers. Regurgitation usually occurs in late infancy, but there is a weak relationship with GERD that occurs later in life. For example, frequent regurgitation in infancy and GERD in the mother (not the father) are risk factors that increase the occurrence of reflux-related symptoms in childhood [14]. In addition, it has been shown in a recent study that the psychopathological personality traits of the mother negatively affect the baby's eating behavior and are effective in the development of reflux [15].

In a prospective study, it was found that babies with frequent vomiting more than 90 days in the first 2 years of life showed more adult symptoms of reflux at the age of 8–9 years [16].

4. Pathophysiology

The lower esophageal sphincter forms a functional barrier between the stomach and the esophagus and prevents the retrograde passage of stomach contents (acid, pepsin, sometimes bile) to the esophagus [17]. In addition, factors facilitating gastroesophageal reflux in CHD infants are the following:

1. Antireflux barrier dysfunction

2. Inadequate clearance mechanism of the esophagus

3. Impairment of esophageal mucosal resistance

4. Delay in gastric emptying

4.1 Antireflux barrier dysfunction

The physiological structure formed by the circular muscles, diaphragm cruses, and phrenoesophageal ligament in the esophagogastric junction forms the lower esopha-geal sphincter (LES) which acts as the primary barrier function for reflux. In addition, the His angle between the esophagus and fundus and the intraabdominal segment of the esophagogastric junction are other components of the antireflux barrier.

The main problem leading to primary gastroesophageal reflux is not the loose of the lower esophageal sphincter; it is known that there are transient relaxations lasting longer than 5 seconds, independent of swallowing [17, 18]. Also some hormones (cholecystokinin, glucagon, vasoactive intestinal peptide (VIP), nitric oxide (NO), dopamine, secretin, and estrogen), drugs (atropine), and nutrients (peppermint, and cocoa) may contribute to GERD by reducing LES pressure [17]. In addition, the presence of stress associated with intensive treatment periods and interventions in complicated CHD patients may lead to increased catecholamine levels. Therefore, it may increase the expression of acid secretion and cause reflux formation [19].

4.2 Inadequate clearance mechanism of the esophagus

Physiological reflux attacks return the secretions and nutrients that escaped from the stomach to the esophagus for a very short period of time with the effect of normal esophageal peristalsis and gravity. In this way, acid, pepsin, and bile which may cause inflammation when it comes into contact with the esophageal mucosa are removed. However, the acid which has not been cleared from the esophageal mucosa is neutralized by swallowing saliva at the alkaline pH. The aim is to remove the gastric contents that will cause inflammation in the esophageal mucosa. Disruption of these natural mechanisms increases the exposure to reflux [20].

4.3 Impairment of esophageal mucosal resistance

The mucus layer and bicarbonate concentration covering the esophageal epithelium, the connections between epithelial cell membrane and cells, intra- and extracellular buffers, blood flow at the postepithelial level, and acid-base balance in the tissue are the factors that provide the resistance of the esophageal mucosa.

4.4 Delay in gastric emptying

Breast milk is known to have a healing effect on the intestinal mucosa and is well absorbed from the mucosa. However, it cannot provide sufficient energy support alone in infants with CHD. Therefore, high-energy density formulas used in patients receiving nutritional support due to increased energy support cause reflux by delaying gastric emptying. Increased fluid and sodium load, especially in patients with heart failure, increases the existing failure and therefore leads to malnutrition and increased metabolic consumption. In the presence of hepatomegaly and ascites, gastric emptying is delayed due to the compression of the stomach, and this delay causes gastroesophageal reflux [3, 21, 22].

Impaired gastrointestinal motility, the presence of protein-losing enteropathy, and the presence of mucosal atrophy secondary to decreased splanchnic blood flow significantly slow the frequency of food elimination and gastric emptying in infants with CHD [1, 4]. Heart failure, especially in infants with critical congenital heart disease, causes some gastrointestinal problems in addition to the findings of the present disease. It causes intestinal edema, malabsorption, steatorrhea, and protein-losing enteropathy, which cause malnutrition. If the clinical situation cannot be controlled and progresses, it forms the basis for gastroesophageal reflux disease [4, 10, 23].

Animasahun et al. reported in their study that cyanosis was the most common presentation of congenital heart disease in children [14]. In a survey based on the frequency of GERD in CHD infants, cyanosis was found to be more frequent in favor of reflux in the group with cyanotic CHD. However, it was stated that this finding is not specific for reflux in CHD infants because this may also be caused by disease [10].

As a result insufficiency of lower esophageal sphincter, transient LES loosening, deterioration of esophageal dysmotility and esophageal clearance, stress and hormonal factors that increase gastric acidity, as well as delayed emptying of the stomach and using high-energy density formulas play a role in reflux pathophysiology of CHD patients.

5. Clinical presentations

A thorough history, a detailed physical examination, and warning symptoms to exclude differential diagnoses are sufficient to make a clinical diagnosis of uncomplicated infant reflux. Regurgitation is the most frequent symptoms of infantile gastroesophageal reflux. In contrast to gastroesophageal reflux that occurs after birth, regurgitation may not be pronounced until the second or third week of life. The typical symptom of physiological reflux is effortless and painless regurgitation

Alarm symptoms in a vomiting baby	
Presence of bile	Diarrhea
Gastrointestinal bleeding	Fever
Presence of force vomiting	Lethargy
Failure to thrive	Hepatosplenomegaly
Presence of blood	Bulging fontanel
Abdominal distension	Macro/microcephaly
	Seizure
	Suspected genetic/metabolic syndrome

Table 2.
Alarm symptoms requiring further investigation in infants with regurgitation and vomiting.

which is called "happy spitter" [24]. A detailed nutritional history including the frequent amount of vomiting and regurgitation, feeding type (breastfeeding or formula), turning blue/purple in feeding time, hiccups, and behavior of the baby during feeding should be obtained.

In order to protect the airway from reflux during infancy, the dystonic posture formed by throwing back the baby's head and sometimes the body can be mistakenly perceived as "seizure." This condition, known as "Sandifer syndrome," protects the airways from reflux or reduces abdominal pain caused by acid reflux. This position regresses with antireflux therapy [25, 26].

Unexplained crying attacks and restless behaviors during the day are associated with various conditions in infants. Healthy infants have crying attacks and restlessness on an average between 0 and 2 hours during the day. Excessive crying attacks and increased restlessness expressed by the family should be considered [27]. Feranchak and colleagues showed during video and pH monitoring study that infants had excessive crying attacks during reflux episodes [28].

Regurgitation, vomiting, irritability, and refusal of feeding which are common in infants may be clinical signs of reflux although food allergies that may develop with the same clinical presentation especially in infant children should be included in the differential diagnosis. Remember that vomiting/regurgitation during infancy may be the first sign of systemic infection, sepsis, or many metabolic diseases other than reflux [29]. Alarm symptoms should be questioned, especially in infants with vomiting under 1 year of age (**Table 2**).

6. Diagnosis

The first step in making a definitive diagnosis in gastroesophageal reflux disease is to suspect. The findings should be questioned with careful and detailed history. Anamnesis and physical examination are the basis of the treatment. A specific diagnostic test is not required to diagnose reflux in the presence of recurrent postprandial vomiting with typical history, especially in infants under 1 year of age. However, if symptoms are not typical or if reflux-related complications are suspected, specific methods should be used. Many methods are used for the diagnosis of GER. Each of these methods is important in obtaining different information [10, 30–32].

6.1 Surveys

The diagnosis of GERD in adults can generally be made by anamnesis and clinical history [33]. Since the complaints are difficult to identify in children under

12 years of age, the history is less reliable [34, 35]. The questionnaire forms are aimed at increasing the reliability of the history rather than making the diagnosis. It is widely accepted surveys that I-GERQ-R developed by Orenstein et al. and GSQ-I and GSQ-YC prepared by Deal et al. could be used in infants with gastroesophageal reflux [10, 35–37].

6.2 Barium contrast radiography

An upper gastrointestinal (GI) series are not sensitive and specific for the diagnosis of GERD. Especially in studies comparing esophageal pH studies, sensitivity, specificity, and positive predictive values were found to be very low [38, 39]. Therefore, radiological evaluation is not an appropriate method to confirm or exclude GERD. However, it can be used especially in the evaluation of selected cases with atypical or severe symptoms such as dysphagia or odynophagia. In these patients provides recognition of anatomical disorders such as achalasia, tracheoesophageal fistula, esophageal stricture, hiatal hernia, antral web, pyloric stenosis, intestinal malrotation or peptic strictures [33, 39].

6.3 Nuclear scintigraphy

Nuclear scintigraphy is a method of demonstrating the spread of isotope in the esophagus, stomach, and lung by ingestion of technetium-labeled food or food. The potential advantage when compared with the esophageal pH study is that it also shows reflux of nonacidic gastric contents and determines gastric emptying rate [40, 41]. However, its sensitivity and specificity are lower than the pH study. Therefore, its place in the diagnosis of GERD is limited and is not routinely recommended [24, 42].

6.4 Esophageal pH monitoring

The important advantages of 24 hr monitoring that can show the relationship between GERD and the patient's symptoms and allow the baby to be monitored for a long time (night, day, according to the position of the body) in the physiological environment [5]. It is used frequently in the diagnosis of patients with non-gastrointestinal symptoms (such as stridor, cough, hoarseness, chest pain) and in the evaluation of the response to medical treatment in patients with refractory gastroesophageal reflux [43, 44].

24 hr monitoring in esophagitis shows the duration, frequency of acidic reflux, and the degree of pH to which the esophagus is exposed [45]. Since it is a useful method in finding and evaluating reflux, it is widely accepted as the gold standard [43, 46, 47]. However, problems such as breast milk shifting the pH of the stomach to the alkaline side, the amount of reflux cannot be determined, and the pH probe cannot be fully inserted into the lower end of the esophagus are disadvantages of this method [45, 47].

6.5 Endoscopic evaluation

Esophageal endoscopy and biopsy are other valuable methods for the diagnosis of GERD. Endoscopy is used to diagnose complications such as erosive esophagitis, stricture, and Barrett's esophagus. Esophageal biopsy can be used in the histological diagnosis of reflux esophagitis in the absence of erosion and in the differentiation of allergic and infection-induced esophagitis. It also helps to exclude diseases such as allergic or infectious esophagitis.

The normal appearance of the esophagus on endoscopy does not exclude histopathological esophagitis. Minimal mucosal changes such as erythema and pallor may occur without esophagitis [48]. In one study, 87% of 62 patients with esophagitis had normal or mild mucosal changes endoscopically [49]. There are no eosinophils and neutrophils in the esophageal epithelium in healthy infants and children [50]. Intraepithelial eosinophilia, which is one of the diagnostic criteria for reflux esophagitis, shows that the esophagus is associated with long-term reflux injury [51].

7. Treatment

Physiological reflux should be considered in the approach to gastroesophageal reflux for infants with congenital heart disease, and patients should be followed up closely (1–2 month periods). Treatment decisions should be made according to the current clinical situation and follow-up [10]. GERD treatment in infants consists of three main topics.

1. Conservative measures

2. Pharmacological treatment

3. Surgical treatment

7.1 Conservative measures

7.1.1 Lifestyle changes

Lifestyle changes or regulation may vary according to age in infants, young children, and older children/adolescents. However, what is known is that lifestyle changes are effective in the prevention of GERD in infants as well as in adults. Education of parents and awareness raising of reflux, nutritional and positional changes are involved in the management of physiological reflux [52–54]. Lifestyle changes in non-pathological reflux should be made before aggressive treatment approaches in infants with CHD such as healthy infants [10].

7.1.2 Positioning

Antireflux conservative measures recommended during infancy are not to feed the baby in a supine position, to allow time to release gas for decompression of the stomach in the middle of the feeding, to place the baby in an anti-Trendelenburg position at 30° after feeding, and not to allow constipation [54, 55]. Many studies have shown that infants lying in the prone position significantly reduce acid reflux compared to the flat supine position [56]. Although keeping the head higher in the prone position was found to reduce reflux further, no such difference was found in the supine position. Despite its positive effect on prevention of reflux, finding a relationship between prone position and sudden infant death prevented this method to be recommended. However, if the child is still observed, this position can be applied after feeding [57, 58].

7.1.3 Dietary change

Since breast-fed infants are less likely to have GERD than infants who take formula, the importance of breastfeeding should be explained and encouraged them. In this age group, cow's milk allergy symptoms (regurgitation, vomiting, sometimes refusal to feed, and restlessness) may not be distinguished from physiological reflux [59–61]. Therefore, in infants with persistent reflux symptoms, cow milk elimination should be performed for 2–3 weeks, and the patient should be followed up. The significant reduction in vomiting and other symptoms during this period and recurrence of symptoms when the diet is impaired suggest cow's milk allergy [62].

It has been shown that the thickening of formulas and nutrients prevents weight loss by reducing vomiting and regurgitation rather than reflux episodes. For this purpose, adding the products containing thickeners (rice cereal, corn or potato starch, and carob bean gum) to thickeners may reduce the frequency and volume of regurgitation [63].

7.2 Pharmacological treatment

Pharmacotherapy therapy is not indicated in infants with CHD who has uncomplicated gastroesophageal reflux because physiological reflux tends to improve over time. Pharmacotherapy should be considered in the treatment of gastroesophageal reflux disease in patients who do not respond despite thickened feedings, lifestyle changes, and nutritional recommendations [64, 65].

7.2.1 Proton pump inhibitors

This group prevents acid secretion by inhibiting Na^+ - K^+ ATPase, called proton pump, which is responsible for acid secretion in parietal cells. Proton pump inhibitors, which have a stronger acid suppressant and mucosal curative effect than H2RAs, maintain gastric pH above 4 and inhibit food-borne acid secretion. It is also more effective in healing erosive esophagitis. It is also more effective in healing erosive esophagitis. Their efficacy is 24 hours, so they have the advantage of using a single dose per day. Proton pump inhibitors, omeprazole, lansoprazole, and esomeprazole, which can be used in the treatment of infants with gastroesophageal reflux, should be appropriately adjusted: omeprazole (infants: 3–<5 kg, 2.5 mg/day; 5–<10 kg, 5 mg/day; ≥10 kg, 10 mg/day), esomeprazole (infants: 3–<5 kg, 2.5 mg/day; 5–<10 kg, 5 mg/day; ≥10 kg, 10 mg/day), and lansoprazole (infants and children: 1 mg/kg/day [maximum 15 mg/day]) [38, 65].

There are potential risks of acid suppression due to PPI treatment in young children, which can be evaluated in four categories: idiosyncratic reactions, drug-drug interactions, drug-induced hypergastrinemia, and drug-induced hypochlorhydria [66]. The most common idiosyncratic reactions were detected in 14% of children receiving PPI and showed effects such as headache, diarrhea, constipation, and nausea. They can be improved by reducing the dose or replacing it with a different preparation [67, 68].

7.2.2 H₂ receptor antagonists

The mechanism of action of H_2 receptor antagonists, which is mainly used in children under 1 year of age, is to reduce acid secretion by inhibiting histamine 2 receptors in gastric parietal cells [53, 66]. Cimetidine, ranitidine, nizatidine, and famotidine are drugs in this group used in the treatment of reflux esophagitis. The frequency and dosage of use of these drugs in children are as follows: cimetidine (children: 30–40 mg/kg/day divided into four doses); ranitidine (children: 5–10 mg/kg/day divided into two to three doses), which is the most preferred drug in the treatment of infants and children; famotidine (children: 1 mg/kg/day divided into two doses); and nizatidine (children: 10–20 mg/kg/day divided into two doses) [38]. Although H2 receptor antagonists reduce pepsin and gastric acid secretion, they do not reduce the frequency of gastroesophageal reflux and are less effective than proton pump inhibitors.

If they are used in reflux treatment for a long time (>14 days), tachyphylaxis and hypochlorhydria which can lead to bacterial colonization may occur. Common adverse events include increased risk of enteritis infection, especially *C. difficile* enteritis, drowsiness, dizziness, headache, abdominal pain, and diarrhea [69–71].

7.2.3 Antacids

The mechanism of action of antacids containing a combination of magnesium, aluminum hydroxide, or calcium carbonate is shown by neutralizing gastric acid. The use of aluminum-containing antacids in infants can cause osteopenia, microcytic anemia, and neurotoxicity, so it is not suitable for use in infants [72].

7.2.4 Surface barrier agents

Alginate and sucralfate are used as surface protection agents in reflux treatment [24, 73]. According to the results of the meta-analysis in 2017, alginates have been shown to be less effective than H2 receptor antagonists and proton pump inhibitors. Alginates are water-soluble salts of alginic acid and act as protective agents for the mucosal surface. Sodium and magnesium alginate preparations have been shown to significantly reduce vomiting symptoms even in preterm and term infants by pH/MMI studies [74]. Sucralfate, composed of sucrose sulfate aluminum, converts into a gel form with gastric acid and adheres to the mucosa, which is exposed to peptic erosion. Its efficacy has been shown in children in a limited number of studies, but there are not enough studies in terms of its efficacy and side effects and safety [75, 76].

7.2.5 Prokinetic agents

Metoclopramide, cisapride, domperidone, and baclofen are among the drugs in this group and can be used in the treatment of gastroesophageal reflux disease. However, cohort studies have shown that prokinetic drugs are not helpful in treatment of reflux [77]. In addition, these agents are not recommended for use in infants and children as they have important side effects such as lethargy, irritability, gynecomastia, galactorrhea, ventricular arrhythmias, QT prolongation, extrapyramidal reactions, and persistent tardive dyskinesia [78, 79].

7.3 Surgical treatment

Surgical procedures such as fundoplication (Nissen) are rarely performed under 1 year of age for indications such as recurrent pneumonia and life-threatening reactive airway disease. It is a method that can be applied in the case of cardiopulmonary insufficiency, which is unresponsive to medical treatment in patients with CHD [80, 81].

Conflicts of interest and sources of funding

The authors disclose that they received no financial support for this work. The authors declare no conflict of interest.

Author details

Mehmet Semih Demirtaş
Aksaray University Education and Research Hospital, Department of Pediatrics,
Turkey

*Address all correspondence to: md.semihdemirtas@gmail.com

IntechOpen

References

[1] Bernstein D. Congenital heart disease. In: Behrman RE, Kliegman RM, Jenson HB, editors. Nelson Textbook of Pediatrics. 17th ed. United States of America: Saunders; 2004. pp. 1499-1554

[2] Özkutlu S, Günal N. Türkiye'de doğumsal kalp hastalıkları prevelansı, tanıdaki sosyoekonomik ve kültürel problemler yeni tanı metotlarının uygulanabilirliği çözümler. Türkiye Klinikleri Kardiyoloji. 2003;4(16):369-371

[3] Costello CL, Gellatly M, Daniel J, Justo RN, Weir K. Growth restriction in infants and young children with congenital heart disease. Congenital Heart Disease. 2015;10(5):447-456

[4] Kuwata S, Iwamoto Y, Ishido H, Taketadu M, Tamura M, Senzaki H. Duodenal tube feeding: An alternative approach for effectively promoting weight gain in children with gastroesophageal reflux and congenital heart disease. Gastroenterology Research and Practice. 2013;2013:181604

[5] Leung AK. Gastroesophageal reflux. In: Leung AK, editor. Common Problems in Ambulatory Pediatrics: Specific Clinical Problems. Vol. 1. New York, NY: Nova Science Publishers, Inc.; 2011. pp. 7-13

[6] Winter HS. Management of Gastroesophageal Reflux Disease in Children and Adolescents. In: Post TW, ed. UpToDate. Waltham, MA [Accessed: 01 April 2019]

[7] Forbes D, Lim A, Ravikumara M. Gastroesophageal reflux in the 21st century. Current Opinion in Pediatrics. 2013;25(5):597-603. DOI: 10.1097/MOP.0b013e328363ecf5

[8] Nelson SP, Chen EH, Syniar GM, et al. Prevalence of symptomatic gastroesophageal reflux during infancy.

A pediatric practice-based survey, pediatric practice research group. Archives of Pediatrics & Adolescent Medicine. 1997;151:569-572

[9] De S, Rajeshwari K, Kalra KK, et al. Gastroesophageal reflux in infants and children in North India. Tropical Gastroenterology. 2001;22:99-102

[10] Demirtaş MS, Karakurt C, Selimoğlu A, Bağ HGG. Is gastroesophageal reflux disease a common complication in infants with congenital heart disease? Turkiye Klinikleri Journal of Pediatrics. 2019;28(1):19-27. DOI: 10.5336/pediatr.2018-63316

[11] El-Serag HB, Gilger M, Carter J, et al. Childhood GERD is a risk factor for GERD in adolescents and young adults. The American Journal of Gastroenterology. 2004;99:806-812

[12] Winter HS, Illueca M, Henderson C, Vaezi M. Review of the persistence of gastroesophageal reflux disease in children, adolescents and adults: Does gastroesophageal reflux disease in adults sometimes begin in childhood? Scandinavian Journal of Gastroenterol. Oct 2011;46(10):1157-1168. DOI: 10.3109/00365521.2011.591425

[13] Orenstein SR, Shalaby TM, Finch R, et al. Autosomal dominant infantile gastroesophageal reflux disease: Exclusion of a 13q14 locus in five well-characterized families. The American Journal of Gastroenterology. 2002;97(11):2725-2732

[14] Animasahun BA, Madise-Wobo AD, Kusimo OY. Cyanotic congenital heart diseases among Nigerian children. Cardiovascular Diagnosis and Therapy. 2017;7:389-396

[15] Karacetin G, Demir T, Erkan T, Cokugras FC. Maternal psychopathology

and psychomotor development of children with gastroesophageal reflux disease. Journal of Pediatric Gastroenterology and Nutrition. Oct 2011;**53**(4):380-385. DOI: 10.1097/ MPG.0b013e3182298caa

[16] Martin AJ, Pratt N, Kennedy JD, et al. Natural history and familial relationships of infant spilling to 9 years of age. Pediatrics. 2002;**109**:1061-1067

[17] Rubenstein JH, Chen JW. Epidemiology of gastroesophageal reflux disease. Gastroenterology Clinics of North America. 2014;**43**(1):1-14

[18] Carroll MW, Jacobson K. Gastroesophageal reflux disease in children and adolescents: When and how to treat. Paediatric Drugs. 2012;**14**(2):79-89

[19] Arad-Cohen N, Cohen A, Tirosh E. The relationship between gastroesophageal reflux and apnea in infants. The Journal of Pediatrics. 2000;**137**(3):321-326

[20] Orlanco RC. Pathophysiology of gastroesophageal reflux disease. In: Castell DO, Richter JE, editors. The Esophagus. 3rd ed. Philadelphia: Lippincott, Williams and Wilkins; 1999. pp. 409-419

[21] Medoff-Cooper B, Ravishankar C. Nutrition and growth in congenital heart disease: A challenge in children. Current Opinion in Cardiology. 2013;**28**(2):122-129

[22] Cribbs RK, Heiss KF, Clabby ML, Wulkan ML. Gastric fundoplication is effective in promoting weight gain in children with severe congenital heart defects. Journal of Pediatric Surgery. 2008;**43**(2):283-289

[23] Schumacher KR, Yu S, Butts R, et al. Fontan-associated protein-losing enteropathy and post–heart transplant outcomes: A multicenter study.

The Journal of Heart and Lung Transplantation. 2019;**38**(1):17-25. DOI: 10.1016/j.healun.2018.09.024

[24] Vandenplas Y, Rudolph CD, Di Lorenzo C, et al. Pediatric gastroesophageal reflux clinical practice guidelines: Joint recommendations of the North American Society for Pediatric Gastroenterology, Hepatology, and Nutrition (NASPGHAN) and the European Society for Pediatric Gastroenterology, Hepatology, and Nutrition. Journal of Pediatric Gastroenterology and Nutrition. 2009;**49**(4):498-547

[25] Frankel EA, Shalaby TM, Orenstein SR. Sandifer syndrome posturing: Relation to abdominal wall contractions, gastroesophageal reflux, and fundoplication. Digestive Diseases and Sciences. 2006;**51**:635-640

[26] Kotagal P, Costa M, Wyllie E, Wolgamuth B. Paroxysmal nonepileptic events in children adolescents. Pediatrics. 2002;**110**:46

[27] Khan S, Orenstein SR. Gastroesophageal reflux disease in infants and children. In: Granderath FA, Kamolz T, Pointner R, editors. Gastroesophageal Reflux Disease. New York: Springer; 2006. pp. 45-64

[28] Feranchak AP, Orenstein SR, Cohn JF. Behaviors associated with onset of gastroesophageal reflux episodes in infants: Prospective study using split-screen video and pH probe. La Clinica Pediatrica. 1994;**33**:654-662

[29] Hegar B, Vandenplas Y. Gastroesophageal reflux: Natural evolution, diagnostic approach and treatment. The Turkish Journal of Pediatrics. 2013;**55**(1):1-7

[30] Rosen R. Gastroesophageal reflux in infants: More than just a phenomenon. JAMA Pediatrics. 2014;**168**(1):83-89. DOI: 10.1001/jamapediatrics.2013.2911

[31] Sullivan JS, Sundaram SS. Gastroesophageal reflux. Pediatrics in Review. 2012;**33**(6):243-253; quiz 254. DOI: 10.1542/pir.33-6-243

[32] Sarath Kumar KS, Mungara J, Venumbaka NR, Vijayakumar P, Karunakaran D. Oral manifestations of gastroesophageal reflux disease in children: A preliminary observational study. Journal of the Indian Society of Pedodontics and Preventive Dentistry. 2018;**36**(2):125-129. DOI: 10.4103/JISPPD.JISPPD_1182_17

[33] Rosen R, Vandenplas Y, Singendonk M, et al. Pediatric Gastroesophageal Reflux Clinical Practice Guidelines: Joint Recommendations of the North American Society for Pediatric Gastroenterology, Hepatology, and Nutrition (NASPGHAN) and the European Society for Pediatric Gastroenterology, Hepatology, and Nutrition (ESPGHAN). Journal of Pediatric Gastroenterology and Nutrition. 25 Jan 2018. DOI: 10.1097

[34] Salvia G, De Vizia B, Manguso F. Effect of intragastric volume and osmolality on mechanisms of gastroesophageal reflux in children with gastroesophageal reflux disease. The American Journal of Gastroenterology. 2001;**96**:1725-1732

[35] Kleinman L, Revicki DA, Flood E. Validation issues in questionnaires for diagnosis and monitoring of gastroesophageal reflux disease in children. Current Gastroenterology Reports. 2006;**8**:230-236

[36] Orenstein SR, Cohn JF, Shalaby T. Reliability and validity of an infant gastroesophageal questionnaire. La Clinica Pediatrica. 1993;**32**:472-484

[37] Deal L, Gold BD, Gremse DA, Winter HS, et al. Age-specific questionnaires distinguish GERD symptom frequency and severity in bebeks and young children: Development and initial validation.

Journal of Pediatric Gastroenterology and Nutrition. 2005;**41**:178-185

[38] Winter HS. Gastroesophageal Reflux in Infants. In: Post TW, ed. UpToDate. Waltham, MA [Accessed: 01 April 2019]

[39] Chen MY, Ott DJ, Sinclair JW, et al. Gastroesophageal reflux disease: Correlation of esophageal pH testing and radiographic findings. Radiology. 1992;**185**:483

[40] Seibert JJ, Byrne WJ, Euler AR, et al. Gastroesophageal reflux—The acid test: Scintigraphy or the pH probe? AJR. American Journal of Roentgenology. 1983;**140**:1087-1090

[41] Fawcett HD, Hayden CK, Adams JC, Swischuk LE. How useful is gastroesophageal reflux scintigraphy in suspected childhood aspiration? Pediatric Radiology. 1988;**18**:311-313

[42] Abell TL, Camilleri M, Donohoe K, et al. Consensus recommendations for gastric emptying scintigraphy: A joint report of the American Neurogastroenterology and Motility Society and the Society of Nuclear Medicine. The American Journal of Gastroenterology. 2008;**103**(3):753-763

[43] Jang HS, Lee JS, Lim GY, Choi BG, Choi GH, Park SH. Correlation of color Doppler sonographic findings with pH measurements in gastroesophageal reflux in children. Journal of Clinical Ultrasound. 2001;**29**(4):212-217. DOI: 10.1002/jcu.1022

[44] van der Pol RJ, Smits MJ, Venmans L, Boluyt N, Benninga MA, Tabbers MM. Diagnostic accuracy of tests in pediatric gastroesophageal reflux disease. The Journal of Pediatrics. 2013;**162**(5):983.e1-987.e4. DOI: 10.1016/j.jpeds.2012.10.041

[45] Lupu VV, Burlea M, Nistor N, et al. Correlation between esophageal

pH-metry and esophagitis in gastroesophageal reflux disease in children. Medicine (Baltimore). 2018;**97**(37):e12042. DOI: 10.1097/MD.0000000000012042

[46] Shay S. Esophageal impedance monitoring: The ups and downs of a new test. The American Journal of Gastroenterology. 2004;**99**(6):1020-1022

[47] Vardar R, Keskin M. Indications of 24-h esophageal pH monitoring, capsule pH monitoring, combined pH monitoring with multichannel impedance, esophageal manometry, radiology and scintigraphy in gastroesophageal reflux disease? The Turkish Journal of Gastroenterology. 2017;**28**(Suppl 1):S16-S21. DOI: 10.5152/tjg.2017.06

[48] Martin R, Hibbs AM. Gastroesophageal Reflux in Premature Infants. In: Post TW, ed. UpToDate. Waltham, MA [Accessed: 01 April 2019]

[49] Black DD, Haggitt RC, Orenstein SR, et al. Esophagitis in infants. Morphometric histological diagnosis and correlation with measure of gastroesophageal reflux. Gastroenterology. 1990;**98**:1408-1414

[50] Tytgat G, Tytgat S. Esophageal biopsy. In: Scarpignato C, Galmiche J-P, editors. Functional Investigation in Esophageal Disease. Basel: Karger; 1994. pp. 13-26

[51] Lightdale JR, Gremse DA. Gastroesophageal reflux: Management guidance for the pediatrician. Pediatrics. 2013;**13**(5):e1684-e1695

[52] Abu Jawdeh EG, Martin RJ. Neonatal apnea and gastroesophageal reflux (GER): Is there a problem? Early Human Development. 2013;**89**(Suppl 1):S14-S16. DOI: 10.1016/S0378-3782(13)70005-7

[53] Rostas SE, McPherson C. Acid suppression for gastroesophageal reflux disease in infants. Neonatal Network. 2018;**37**(1):33-41. DOI: 10.1891/0730-0832.37.1.33

[54] Shalaby TM, Orenstein SR. Efficacy of telephone teaching of conservative therapy for infants with symptomatic gastroesophageal reflux referred by pediatricians to pediatric gastroenterologist. The Journal of Pediatrics. 2003;**142**:57-61

[55] Meyers WF, Herbst JJ. Effectiveness of positioning therapy for gastroesophageal reflux. Pediatrics. 1982;**62**:768-772

[56] Tobin JM, McCloud P, Cameron DJ. Posture and gastro-esophageal reflux: A case for left lateral positioning. Archives of Disease in Childhood. 1997;**76**:254-258

[57] Corvaglia L, Rotatori R, Ferlini M, et al. The effect of body positioning on gastroesophageal reflux in premature infants: Evaluation by combined impedance and pH monitoring. The Journal of Pediatrics. 2007;**151**:591-596

[58] Kaltenbach T, Crockett S, Gerson LB. Are lifestyle measures effective in patients with gastroesophageal reflux disease? An evidence-based approach. Archives of Internal Medicine. 2006;**166**:965-971

[59] Borrelli O, Mancini V, Thapar N, et al. Cow's milk challenge increases weakly acidic reflux in children with cow's milk allergy and gastroesophageal reflux disease. The Journal of Pediatrics. 2012;**161**(3):476-481.e1. DOI: 10.1016/j.jpeds.2012.03.002

[60] Nielsen RG, Bindslev-Jensen C, Kruse-Andersen S, Husby S. Severe gastroesophageal reflux disease and cow milk hypersensitivity in infants and children: disease association and

evaluation of a new challenge procedure. Journal of Pediatric Gastroenterology and Nutrition. 2004;**39**(4):383-391. PubMed PMID: 15448429

[61] Vandenplas Y, Gottrand F, Veereman-Wauters G, et al. Gastrointestinal manifestations of cow's milk protein allergy and gastrointestinal motility. Acta Paediatrica. 2012;**101**(11):1105-1109. DOI: 10.1111/j.1651-2227.2012.02808.x

[62] Campanozzi A, Boccia G, Pensabene L, et al. Prevalence and natural history of gastroesophageal reflux: Pediatric prospective survey. Pediatrics. 2009;**123**(3):779-783. DOI: 10.1542/peds.2007-3569

[63] Horvath A, Dziechciarz P, Szajewska H. The effect of thickened feed interventions on gastroesophageal reflux in infants: Systematic review and meta-analysis of randomized, controlled trials. Pediatrics. 2008;**122**:e1268-e1277

[64] Gibbons TE, Gold BD. The use of proton pump inhibitors in children: A comprehensive review. Paediatric Drugs. 2003;**5**:25-40

[65] Romano C, Chiaro A, Comito D, et al. Proton pump inhibitors in pediatrics: Evaluation of efficacy in GERD therapy. Current Clinical Pharmacology. 2011;**6**:41-47

[66] Mattos ÂZ, Marchese GM, Fonseca BB, Kupski C, Machado MB. Antisecretory treatment for pediatric gastroesophageal reflux disease—A systematic review. Arquivos de Gastroenterologia. 2017;**54**(4):271-280. DOI: 10.1590/s0004-2803.201700000-42

[67] Hassall E, Kerr W, El-Serag HB Characteristics of children receiving proton pump inhibitors continuously for up to 11 years duration. The Journal of Pediatrics. 2007;**150**:262-267

[68] Turco R, Martinelli M, Miele E, et al. Proton pump inhibitors as a risk factor for paediatric *Clostridium difficile* infection. Alimentary Pharmacology & Therapeutics. 2010;**31**(7):754-759. DOI: 10.1111/j.1365-2036.2009.04229.x

[69] Adams DJ, Eberly MD, Rajnik M, Nylund CM. Risk factors for community-associated *Clostridium difficile* infection in children. The Journal of Pediatrics. 2017;**186**:105-109. DOI: 10.1016/j.jpeds.2017.03.032

[70] Canani RB, Cirillo P, Roggero P, et al. Therapy with gastric acidity inhibitors increases the risk of acute gastroenteritis and community-acquired pneumonia in children. Pediatrics. 2006;**117**(5):e817-e820. DOI: 10.1542/peds.2005-1655

[71] Freedberg DE, Lamousé-Smith ES, Lightdale JR, Jin Z, Yang YX, Abrams JA. Use of acid suppression medication is associated with risk for *C. difficile* infection in infants and children: A population-based study. Clinical Infectious Diseases. 2015;**61**(6):912-917

[72] Leung AK, Lai PC. Use of metoclopramide for the treatment of gastroesophageal reflux in infants and children. Current Therapeutic Research, Clinical and Experimental. 1984;**36**:911-915

[73] Simon B, Ravelli GP, Goffin H. Sucralfate gel versus placebo in patients with non-erosive gastro-oesophageal reflux disease. Alimentary Pharmacology & Therapeutics. 1996;**10**:441-446

[74] Leiman DA, Riff BP, Morgan S, et al. Alginate therapy is effective treatment for gastroesophageal reflux disease symptoms: A systematic review and meta-analysis. Diseases of the Esophagus. 2017;**30**(2):1-8. DOI: 10.1111/dote.12535

[75] Atasay B, Erdeve O, Arsan S, Türmen T. Effect of sodium alginate on acid gastroesophageal reflux disease in preterm infants: A pilot study. The Journal of Clinical Pharmacology. 2010;**50**:1267-1272. [Epub: 20 May 2010]

[76] Corvaglia L, Aceti A, Mariani E, et al. The efficacy of sodium alginate (Gaviscon) for the treatment of gastro-oesophageal reflux in preterm infants. Alimentary Pharmacology & Therapeutics. 2011;**33**:466-470. [Epub: 15 December 2010]

[77] Tolia V, Calhoun J, Kuhns L, Kauffman RE. Randomized, prospective double-blind trial of metoclopramide and placebo for gastroesophageal reflux in infants. The Journal of Pediatrics. 1989;**115**(1):141-145. PubMed PMID: 2661788

[78] Dalby-Payne JR, Morris AM, Craig JC. Meta-analysis of randomized controlled trials on the benefits and risks of using cisapride for the treatment of gastroesophageal reflux in children. Journal of Gastroenterology and Hepatology. 2003;**18**:196-202

[79] Hibbs AM, Lorch SA. Metoclopramide for the treatment of gastroesophageal reflux disease in infants: A systematic review. Pediatrics. 2006;**118**:746-752

[80] Wakeman DS, Wilson NA, Warner BW. Current status of surgical management of gastroesophageal reflux in children. Current Opinion in Pediatrics. 2016;**28**(3):356-362. DOI: 10.1097/MOP.0000000000000341

[81] Kane TD, Brown MF, Chen MK, et al. Position paper on laparoscopic antireflux operations in infants and children for gastroesophageal reflux disease. American Pediatric Surgery Association. Journal of Pediatric Surgery. 2009;**44**:1034-1040

Chapter 4

Practical Approach to Chest Pain Related to Cardiac Implantable Electronic Device Implantation

Umashankar Lakshmanadoss, Imran Sulemankhil
and Karnika Senthilkumar

Abstract

In this review article, we described the common causes and approach for chest pain that happens after cardiac device implantation surgeries. We also describe the clinical features and appropriate treatment for them.

Keywords: CIED implant, chest pain, pericardial effusion, pneumothorax, erosion of device

1. Introduction

Cardiac implantable electronic devices (CIED) are being implanted for more than 600,000 patients on a yearly basis [1]. These CIEDs include pacemakers, implantable cardioverter defibrillators, and cardiac resynchronization therapy devices [2]. These implantation surgeries are not without risk, as there are many potential complications that can occur either immediately or in a delayed setting [3–6]. Many of the complications could have a common presentation of chest pain, and depending on the etiology, morbidity, and mortality can vary widely [7]. The surgical process itself during the cardiac implantation device surgery can result in chest pain [8]. However, it is paramount to differentiate chest pain due to acute coronary syndrome (ACS) from non-ischemic causes. In the setting of a ventricular paced rhythm or left bundle branch block, this can be difficult with electrocardiography as the ST segments or T waves may hide or mimic ACS [9]. In this situation, the modified Sgarbossa criteria can be implemented to improve the diagnostic accuracy of electrocardiography in this patient population [10–12]. Hence, it is very important to identify the causes of chest pain after any cardiac implantation device surgery. In this chapter, we will discuss a practical approach to chest pain after cardiac implantation device surgery.

2. Chest pain after CIED implantation

For practical purposes, the etiology of chest pain after device implantation surgery could be divided based on the time of occurrence. We classified it into the following three categories:

1. Immediate chest pain (during the procedure)

2. Post procedural chest pain (in the immediate postoperative period, within 1–2 days)

3. Delayed chest pain

Just like any other surgical process, placing the leads and the devices resulted in various forms of trauma and by itself can produce chest pain. These adverse effects can occur during the procedure, in the immediate postoperative period, and well after the implant procedure.

2.1 Immediate chest pain during the procedure

2.1.1 Musculoskeletal

Most of these CIED surgeries are performed with moderate sedation [13]. Patients who undergo CIED surgeries are commonly elderly and have multiple co-morbid conditions [14]. This clearly limits the options for adequate analgesia and sedation due to concerns for adverse effects of sedatives and analgesics. Hence, adequate local anesthesia plays a major role in terms of pain control. If the patients are not adequately anesthetized with local anesthesia, they may experience sharp pain during various parts of device implantation. Even if they are adequately anesthetized with local anesthesia, this will be effective predominantly within the subcutaneous tissue [15]. Furthermore, patients may feel sharp pain when the muscle tissue is being manipulated, especially if they have to have a suture or cauterization of the muscles secondary to inadvertent bleeding. Safe vascular access is very important to minimize the complications of CIED surgery. Hence, most of the operating physicians try to use the junction between the clavicle and first rib as a landmark to minimize the risk of pneumothorax. Typically, the axillary vein can be accessed just at the level of the first rib [16]. If the needle passes the veins "through and through" and hits the periosteum of the first rib, patients may feel this discomfort. After venous access, when the sheath is being advanced into the venous system, it could stretch the periosteum of the costoclavicular ligament which in turn can be uncomfortable for the patient. Hence, during this part of the procedure, it is very important to provide appropriate analgesia for the patient.

2.1.2 Pneumothorax

Pneumothorax, hemothorax, and hydropneumothorax are some of the dangerous complications after CIED implantation [17]. Implanting-physicians always strive to minimize these complications as they increase the morbidity and mortality. These complications are reduced by using micropuncture access needles, using contrast venography to identify the veins, and using ultrasound to identify the veins [18–20]. In addition to this, some physicians also use a bolus of intravenous fluid to engorge veins. Similarly, Trendelenburg positioning or elevating the patient's legs with a wedge under the leg (without tilting the operating table) could be useful [21]. Some physicians also inject contrast when they are gaining access because the contrast tends to engorge the veins. In spite of these careful and meticulous approaches, sometimes pneumothorax is inevitable. Even though, the vein is accessed via the extrathoracic veins, it is possible that the patients may have a small bleb secondary to COPD, which through inadvertent entry may produce a pneumothorax [22]. Pneumothorax could be suspected at the earliest, when there is aspiration of air with the introducer needle, before entering into the venous system. It is also imperative to note that the needle should be attached to the syringe air tight. Otherwise, it could give a false opinion of aspiration of air into the syringe. During access, after entering into the vein, if the patient has obstructive sleep apnea, they could create huge negative intrathoracic pressure during deep inspiration which in turn can suck in air (**Figure 1**).

Causes of pneumothorax:

1. Advancing the needle deep into the lung parenchyma, beyond the first rib

2. Accidental puncture of superficial blebs

3. Medial puncture (intrathoracic part of the subclavian vein)

If the operating physician noted any signs of aspiration of air into the syringe, then the patient should be carefully monitored for possible pneumothorax. In addition to this, patients may also develop sudden onset of chest pain, cough, hypoxia or tachycardia. During this situation, fluoroscopy can be implemented immediately to evaluate for any pneumothorax; keeping in mind that supine positioning is not the ideal method of assessing for pneumothorax.

2.1.3 Mediastinal bleed

Any mediastinal bleed during CIED implantation could produce acute chest pain. This pain is typically very diffuse and radiates toward the posterior aspect of the chest secondary to mediastinal reflection [23, 24]. Patients may manifest tachycardia secondary to sympathetic stimulation and hypotension, depending upon the extent of the blood loss. This is one of the dangerous conditions, which needs to be identified and addressed as soon as possible. Inadvertent access of the subclavian artery could produce mediastinal bleed. Hence, accessing the axillary vein at the

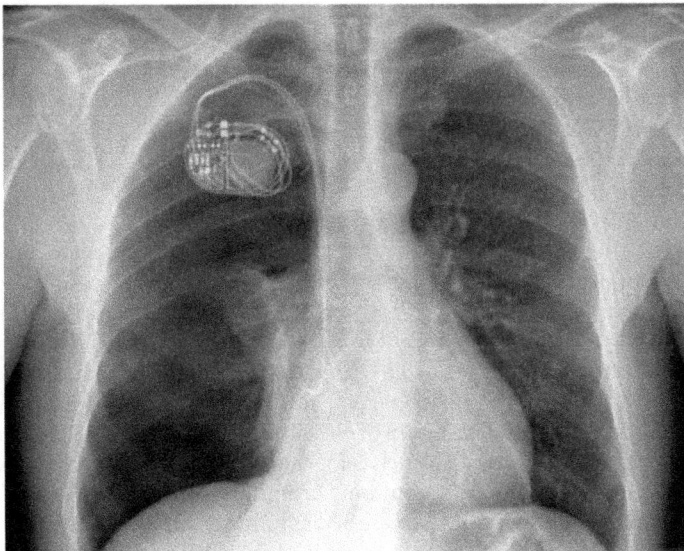

Figure 1.
Chest X-ray showing right sided pneumothorax.

level of the first rib is a preferred approach as it allows for manual compression in this situation [25, 26]. After getting access into the central system, it is very important to advance the guide wire below the diaphragm to confirm placement within the inferior vena cava and not in the arterial side prior to introduction of the sheath. This way, even if there is any inadvertent arterial access, the chances of mediastinal bleeding will be minimized. In the elderly patients, the venous system could be very tortuous especially at the level of the brachiocephalic system [27–29]. Hence, the wire and the sheath have to be advanced very carefully. If there is any resistance noted during advancement of the sheath, further advancement has to be done under fluoroscopic guidance.

2.1.4 Pericardial effusion/tamponade

During device implantation, it is possible that patients may have an acute pericardial bleed leading to either pericardial effusion or pericardial tamponade [17]. Typically, patients have chest pain, tachycardia, and clinical features consistent with cardiogenic shock [30]. Pericardial chest pain typically radiates toward the shoulder blades and also toward the trapezius muscle, at the nape of the neck, due to the pericardial reflection. Further, it may be pleuritic in nature due to rubbing of the pericardium with the pleura [31]. When there is a clinical suspicion for pericardial effusion or pericardial tamponade, immediate imaging is required without any delay; this needs to be addressed immediately, as appropriate treatment is lifesaving. Perforation at the level of the intra-pericardial superior vena cava, right atrium, right atrial appendage, coronary sinus, or right ventricle are all possible and can lead to pericardial effusion [32, 33]. If there is any suspicion of pericardial effusion, immediate fluoroscopic evaluation looking for the lateral movement of the pericardium is useful. Imaging with transthoracic echocardiogram or intracardiac echocardiogram is also of great benefit. Immediate pericardiocentesis will be lifesaving [34]. It is also possible that there may be a slow and progressively worsening pleural effusion, which may not produce any clinical symptoms immediately and patients may present with late pericardial effusion. Minimal or small pericardial effusion could be managed conservatively by following the patient very closely. High dose aspirin, colchicine, and oral corticosteroids can be used to minimize the inflammatory response [31]. However, if there is any hemodynamic compromise, pericardiocentesis is then indicated. Depending on the clinical situation, lead revision may also be indicated (**Figure 2**).

2.2 Intermediate chest pain, during the recovery and within 1–2 days

2.2.1 Surgical site pain

As in any surgical procedure, the most common reason for the pain is usually due to postoperative swelling and will typically respond to simple analgesics and cold compression. In addition to this, it could be due to mechanical reasons including superficial placement of the device within the subcutaneous tissue leading to too much pressure on the skin, lateral device placement in the infraclavicular region leading to mechanical irritation of the axillary nerve, nerve entrapment, etc. [35–37]. Very rarely, patients can also develop allergic reactions to the components of the CIED including titanium, cadmium, chromium, and nickel [38–40]. As these patients are typically advised to use an arm sling, their arm movements can be completely restricted which in turn could lead to shoulder pain [41, 42]; this is similar to early phase of adhesive capsulitis.

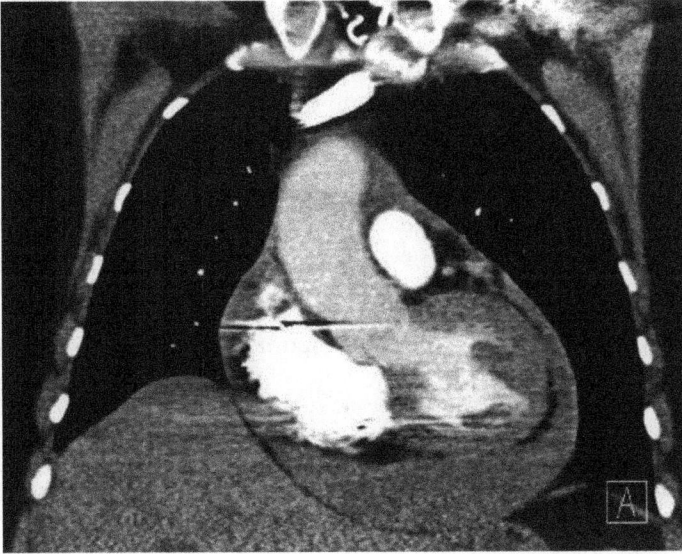

Figure 2.
CT chest showing pericardial effusion.

2.2.2 Pleuritic/pericardial involvement

As discussed above, pneumothorax, pneumopericardium, hydropneumothorax, and pericardial effusion can produce delayed symptoms of pleural or pericardial pain leading to chest pain. This is typically due to a break in the continuity of the pleural or pericardial membrane secondary to lead perforation. It could be secondary to micro or macro perforations [43–45]. Nevertheless, patient symptoms of chest pain have to be evaluated very carefully and investigated accordingly. Simple chest X-ray and transthoracic echocardiogram would be sufficient in most cases [46]. Use of a CT chest could result in overreading lead perforation due to the presence of artifacts [47]. If there is any clinical suspicion for lead dislodgment, in most cases, lead revision would take care of the chest pain immediately.

2.2.3 Stress cardiomyopathy

Patients may develop stress cardiomyopathy/Takotsubo cardiomyopathy, in the postoperative period. Clinically, they may present with chest pain, shortness of breath, new onset arrhythmias, and positive troponins. Transthoracic echocardiogram will show apical ballooning and basal septal sparing [48]. Cardiac catheterization can confirm the absence of any major obstructive coronary artery disease. Even though the pathophysiology of the stress cardiomyopathy is evident, etiology of stress cardiomyopathy in the setting of pacemaker implantation is not very clear. This could be secondary to the stress events which led to the device implantation, medications used for sedation, pacing induced dyssynchrony, and/or due to the stress of the surgical procedure itself [49–51].

2.2.4 Diaphragmatic pacing

In a small percent of the population, it is possible that patients may have diaphragmatic pacing due to direct capture of the phrenic nerve [52]. This can be interpreted as chest discomfort/hiccups, manifesting predominantly in certain position [53]. For a CRT device, the coronary sinus lead would be placed into the posterolateral or lateral branches which would abut the lateral wall of the left ventricle [54, 55]. The left phrenic nerve runs very close toward the lateral border of the left ventricle. Hence, this lead could be pacing the phrenic nerve and producing diaphragmatic contractions. Usually, during lead placement, high output pacing will be performed from the coronary sinus lead to rule out any phrenic nerve capture. However, secondary to displacement of the leads, it is possible that the leads can move and capture the phrenic nerve leading on to diaphragmatic contractions [56]. The right ventricular lead typically does not produce diaphragmatic pacing except in the following situations: (1) perforation of the right ventricle and migration of the lead inferiorly to produce direct capture of the diaphragm; (2) extreme RV dilation to the extent that the lateral border of the cardiac silhouette is situated near the right ventricular apex [57]. These situations require lead revision. On the other hand, the right-sided phrenic nerve travels along the lateral border of the right atrium, distant from the right atrial appendage, and can lead to diaphragmatic pacing if the right atrial lead becomes dislodged and captures the right phrenic nerve [58, 59].

2.3 Delayed onset chest pain

2.3.1 Surgical site pain

In most patients, surgical site chest pain would resolve within a week or so. However, some patients may have prolonged, local chest discomfort secondary to increased sensitivity. Other conditions including superficial device placement leading on to pressure on the skin (usually at the margin of the device), nerve entrapment, hematoma, allergic reactions, erosion, infection, etc., have to be ruled out [35–40]. Depending upon the etiology, we may have to open the pocket again and address the primary reason for the chest pain (**Figure 3**).

2.3.2 Delayed cardiac perforation

Delayed cardiac perforation secondary to CIED leads is uncommon when compared to acute perforation [60–62]. Patients will typically have symptoms of chest pain and the clinical presentation may not be as dramatic as an acute perforation. Hence a high degree of clinical suspicion needs to be maintained and early imaging including X-ray, echocardiogram, and, if needed, CT scan could be beneficial in these patients [62]. Further, device interrogation may show loss of capture, even at high output. Often these patients may need a multi-disciplinary approach including electrophysiologists and cardiothoracic surgeons [63].

2.3.3 Pacemaker-mediated angina

In patients who have underlying coronary artery disease, angina can be precipitated secondary to rapid pacing [64]. Usually, pacemakers are programmed to minimize right ventricular pacing. However, dual-chamber pacemakers tract the atrial electrical activity and the ventricular pacing follows. Hence, in patients with a high sinus rate or atrial tachycardia, the right ventricle could be paced at a higher rate, thereby resulting in demand ischemia [65, 66]. In the setting of underlying clinical or subclinical coronary artery disease, this in turn can lead to angina. This presents as a classical anginal form of chest pain. This can be identified by altering the pacemaker rate. Treatment typically involves reprogramming the device

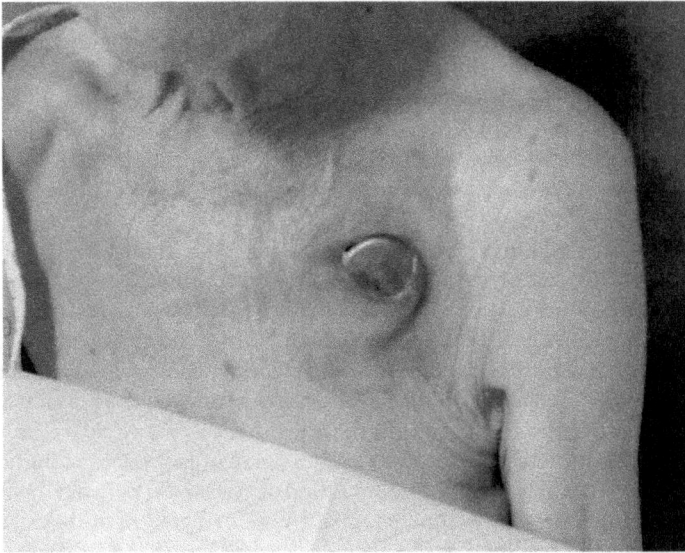

Figure 3.
Cardiac implantable electronic device erosion.

to minimize right ventricular pacing and eventually taking care of the underlying coronary artery disease [67].

2.3.4 Post cardiac injury syndrome

Patients who underwent CRT-D implantation may have a 3–6 week delayed onset of chest pain; this is more pericardial in nature and similar to Dressler syndrome. The main differentiating factor from delayed pericardial effusion/pericardial tamponade is that there is no pericardial fluid in this situation [68]. The pathogenesis of post cardiac injury syndrome is immune mediated. Imazio et al. proposed diagnostic criteria for post cardiac injury syndrome with at least two out of five being required [69].

1. Unexplained fever

2. Pleuritic or pericardial chest pain

3. Pericardial rub on auscultation

4. New or worsening pericardial/pleural effusion on imaging

5. Elevated inflammatory markers including CRP

These patients respond very well to high-dose of aspirin, colchicine, or oral corticosteroids.

2.3.5 Painful left bundle branch block syndrome

Painful left bundle branch block (LBBB) syndrome is one of the uncommon delayed conditions seen with CIED placement [70]. Patients who have right ventricular pacemaker will have left bundle branch block morphology when pacing the right ventricle. On electrocardiography, this can be differentiated from an acute LBBB using the six criteria outlined by Shvilkin et al. [70]: abrupt onset of chest pain coinciding with the development of LBBB; simultaneous resolution of symptoms with resolution of LBBB; normal 12-lead ECGs before and after LBBB; absence of myocardial ischemia during functional stress testing; normal left ventricular function and the absence of other abnormalities to explain symptoms; and low precordial S/T wave ratio consistent with new-onset LBBB (<1.8 in this series) and inferior QRS axis.

Most of the patients tolerate right ventricular pacing without any significant clinical features. However, a small population of patients may develop significant chest pain, independent of coronary artery disease [71, 72]. Although the underlying mechanism is unclear, several mechanisms have been postulated: (1) dyssynchronous ventricular contraction occur due to paradoxical septal movement during ventricular pacing, (2) there is abnormal activation of the neurons responsible for interception ventricular pacing, and (3) there is microvascular ischemia during ventricular pacing as noted by elevated concentration of lactic acid in the coronary sinus [73–75]. A careful history and observation of chest pain only during right ventricular pacing is the clue to the correct diagnosis. Treatment of these patients is very challenging but patients may respond very well to either CRT therapy or His bundle pacing [74, 76–78].

3. Conclusion

Almost all the patients that undergo CIED implantation will have some sort of chest pain dependent on the time of occurrence (**Table 1**). Most of the time this is secondary to surgical site pain. However, this could also be secondary to multiple reasons including life-threatening complications. Hence, early diagnosis and prompt treatment is warranted to minimize morbidity and mortality.

Delayed chest pain	Post procedural chest pain (postoperative period, 1–2 days)	Immediate chest pain (perioperative period)
Surgical site pain	Surgical site pain	Musculoskeletal
Delayed cardiac perforation	Pleuritic/pericardial involvement	Pneumothorax
Pacemaker-mediated angina	Stress cardiomyopathy	Mediastinal bleed
Post cardiac injury syndrome	Diaphragmatic pacing	Pericardial effusion/tamponade
Painful left bundle branch block syndrome		

Table 1.
Chest pain occurrence after cardiac implantable electronic device.

Conflict of interest

The authors declare no conflict of interest.

Author details

Umashankar Lakshmanadoss[1]*, Imran Sulemankhil[2] and Karnika Senthilkumar[3]

1 Mercy Heart Institute, Cincinnati, OH, USA

2 Department of Medicine, Jewish Hospital of Cincinnati, Cincinnati, OH, USA

3 Cambridge International School, Dubai, UAE

*Address all correspondence to: drlumashankar@gmail.com

IntechOpen

References

[1] Wood MA, Ellenbogen KA. Cardiology patient pages. Cardiac pacemakers from the patient's perspective. Circulation. 2002;**105**(18):2136-2138

[2] Steffen MM, Osborn JS, Cutler MJ. Cardiac implantable electronic device therapy: Permanent pacemakers, implantable cardioverter defibrillators, and cardiac resynchronization devices. The Medical Clinics of North America. 2019;**103**(5):931-943

[3] Chauhan A, Grace AA, Newell SA, Stone DL, Shapiro LM, Schofield PM, et al. Early complications after dual chamber versus single chamber pacemaker implantation. Pacing and Clinical Electrophysiology. 1994;**17** (11 Pt 2):2012-2015

[4] Silva KR, Albertini CM, Crevelari ES, Carvalho EI, Fiorelli AI, Martinelli MF, et al. Complications after surgical procedures in patients with cardiac implantable electronic devices: Results of a prospective registry. Arquivos Brasileiros de Cardiologia. 2016;**107**(3):245-256

[5] Blomstrom-Lundqvist C, Traykov V, Erba PA, Burri H, Nielsen JC, Bongiorni MG, et al. European heart rhythm association (EHRA) international consensus document on how to prevent, diagnose, and treat cardiac implantable electronic device infections-endorsed by the heart rhythm society (HRS), the Asia pacific heart rhythm society (APHRS), the Latin American heart rhythm society (LAHRS), international society for cardiovascular infectious diseases (ISCVID) and the European society of clinical microbiology and infectious diseases (ESCMID) in collaboration with the European association for cardio-thoracic surgery (EACTS). Europace. 2020;**22**(4):515-549

[6] Nichols CI, Vose JG. Incidence of bleeding-related complications during primary implantation and replacement of cardiac implantable electronic devices. Journal of the American Heart Association. 2017;**6**(1):e004263. DOI: 10.1161/JAHA.116.004263

[7] Ruigomez A, Rodriguez LA, Wallander MA, Johansson S, Jones R. Chest pain in general practice: Incidence, comorbidity and mortality. Family Practice. 2006;**23**(2):167-174

[8] Biocic M, Vidosevic D, Boric M, Boric T, Giunio L, Fabijanic D, et al. Anesthesia and perioperative pain management during cardiac electronic device implantation. Journal of Pain Research. 2017;**10**:927-932

[9] Sgarbossa EB, Pinski SL, Barbagelata A, Underwood DA, Gates KB, Topol EJ, et al. Electrocardiographic diagnosis of evolving acute myocardial infarction in the presence of left bundle-branch block. GUSTO-1 (global utilization of streptokinase and tissue plasminogen activator for occluded coronary arteries) investigators. The New England Journal of Medicine. 1996;**334**(8):481-487

[10] Smith SW, Dodd KW, Henry TD, Dvorak DM, Pearce LA. Diagnosis of ST-elevation myocardial infarction in the presence of left bundle branch block with the ST-elevation to S-wave ratio in a modified sgarbossa rule. Annals of Emergency Medicine. 2012;**60**(6):766-776

[11] Abraham AS, Vinson DR, Levis JT. ECG diagnosis: Acute myocardial infarction in a ventricular-paced rhythm. The Permanente Journal. 2019;**23**: 19-001. DOI: 10.7812/TPP/19-001

[12] Maloy KR, Bhat R, Davis J, Reed K, Morrissey R. Sgarbossa criteria are

highly specific for acute myocardial infarction with pacemakers. The Western Journal of Emergency Medicine. 2010;**11**(4):354-357

[13] Furniss SS, Sneyd JR. Safe sedation in modern cardiological practice. Heart. 2015;**101**(19):1526-1530

[14] Lim WY, Prabhu S, Schilling RJ. Implantable cardiac electronic devices in the elderly population. Arrhythmia & Electrophysiology Review. 2019;**8**(2):143-146

[15] Becker DE, Reed KL. Essentials of local anesthetic pharmacology. Anesthesia Progress. 2006;**53**(3):98-108

[16] Poole JE, Larson W. Surgical Implantation of Cardiac Rhythm Devices. United States: Elsevier Health Sciences; 2017. pp. 20-25

[17] Aktaa S, Fatania K, Gains C, White H. Chest pain following permanent pacemaker insertion... a case of pneumopericardium due to atrial lead perforation. BML Case Reports. 2018:**2018**. DOI: 10.1136/bcr,2018-226318

[18] Gunda S, Reddy M, Pillarisetti J, Atoui M, Badhwar N, Swarup V, et al. Differences in complication rates between large bore needle and a long micropuncture needle during epicardial access: Time to change clinical practice? Circulation. Arrhythmia and Electrophysiology. 2015;**8**(4):890-895

[19] Seto AH, Abu-Fadel MS, Sparling JM, Zacharias SJ, Daly TS, Harrison AT, et al. Real-time ultrasound guidance facilitates femoral arterial access and reduces vascular complications: FAUST (femoral arterial access with ultrasound trial). JACC. Cardiovascular Interventions. 2010;**3**(7):751-758

[20] Albertini CMM, Silva KRD, Leal Filho JMDM, Crevelari ES, Martinelli Filho M, Carnevale FC, et al. Usefulness of preoperative venography in patients with cardiac implantable electronic devices submitted to lead replacement or device upgrade procedures. Arquivos Brasileiros de Cardiologia. 2018;**111**(5):686-696

[21] Jaroszewski DE, Altemose GT, Scott LR, Srivasthan K, Devaleria PA, Lackey J, et al. Nontraditional surgical approaches for implantation of pacemaker and cardioverter defibrillator systems in patients with limited venous access. The Annals of Thoracic Surgery. 2009;**88**(1):112-116

[22] Kirkfeldt RE, Johansen JB, Nohr EA, Moller M, Arnsbo P, Nielsen JC. Pneumothorax in cardiac pacing: A population-based cohort study of 28,860 Danish patients. Europace. 2012;**14**(8):1132-1138

[23] Scumpia A, Dekok M, Aronovich D, Bajwa G, Barros R, Katz R, et al. Acute chest pain in a patient with a non-strangulated hiatal hernia. Journal of Acute Disease. 2015;**4**(4):344-346

[24] Seo YH, Kwak JY. Spontaneous hemomediastinum and hemothorax caused by a ruptured bronchial artery aneurysm. The Korean Journal of Thoracic and Cardiovascular Surgery. 2011;**44**(4):314-317

[25] Migliore F, Siciliano M, De Lazzari M, Ferretto S, Valle CD, Zorzi A, et al. Axillary vein puncture using fluoroscopic landmarks: A safe and effective approach for implantable cardioverter defibrillator leads. Journal of Interventional Cardiac Electrophysiology. 2015;**43**(3):263-267

[26] Yang F, Kulbak G. A new trick to a routine procedure: Taking the fear out of the axillary vein stick using the 35 degrees caudal view. Europace. 2015;**17**(7):1157-1160

[27] Thomas JB, Antiga L, Che SL, Milner JS, Steinman DA, Spence JD, et al. Variation in the carotid bifurcation geometry of young versus older adults: Implications for geometric risk of atherosclerosis. Stroke. 2005;**36**(11):2450-2456

[28] Lam RC, Lin SC, DeRubertis B, Hynecek R, Kent KC, Faries PL. The impact of increasing age on anatomic factors affecting carotid angioplasty and stenting. Journal of Vascular Surgery. 2007;**45**(5):875-880

[29] Del Corso L, Moruzzo D, Conte B, Agelli M, Romanelli AM, Pastine F, et al. Tortuosity, kinking, and coiling of the carotid artery: Expression of atherosclerosis or aging? Angiology. 1998;**49**(5):361-371

[30] James HA, Wan SH, Wylam ME. Delayed post-operative cardiac tamponade manifesting as cardiogenic shock. Journal of Cardiology Cases. 2013;**8**(6):195-197

[31] Goyle KK, Walling AD. Diagnosing pericarditis. American Family Physician. 2002;**66**(9):1695-1702

[32] Yamada T, Kay GN. In: Huang SKS, Miller JM, editors. Complications Associated with Radiofrequency Catheter Ablation of Arrhythmias. Philadelphia: Content Repository Only! 2019. p. 636. DOI: 10.1016/B978-0-323-52992-1.00038-7

[33] Provaznik Z, Holzamer A, Camboni D, Rupprecht L, Resch M, Wittmann S, et al. Perforation of myocardial wall and great vessels after cardiovascular interventions-a 5-year analysis. The Journal of Thoracic Disease. 2017;**9**(12):5288-5294

[34] American College of Cardiology. 2017. Available from: https://www.acc.org/latest-in-cardiology/articles/2017/10/27/10/20/managing-pericardium-in-electrophysiology-procedures

[35] Jumper N, Radotra I, Witt P, Campbell NG, Mishra A. Brachial plexus impingement secondary to implantable cardioverter defibrillator: A case report. Archives of Plastic Surgery. 2019;**26**:594-598

[36] Harcombe AA, Newell SA, Ludman PF, Wistow TE, Sharples LD, Schofield PM, et al. Late complications following permanent pacemaker implantation or elective unit replacement. Heart. 1998;**80**(3):240-244

[37] Kolker AR, Redstone JS, Tutela JP. Salvage of exposed implantable cardiac electrical devices and lead systems with pocket change and local flap coverage. Annals of Plastic Surgery. 2007;**59**(1):26. Discussion 30

[38] Shittu M, Shah P, Elkhalili W, Suleiman A, Shaaban H, Shah PA, et al. A rare case of recurrent pacemaker allergic reaction. Heart Views. 2015;**16**(2):59-61

[39] Abdallah HI, Balsara RK, O'Riordan AC. Pacemaker contact sensitivity: Clinical recognition and management. The Annals of Thoracic Surgery. 1994;**57**(4):1017-1018

[40] Honari G, Raissi F. Hypersensitivity to cardiovascular implants: Cardiac implantable electronic devices and septal occluders. In: Chen J, Thyssen J, editors. Metal Allergy: From Dermatitis to Implant and Device Failure. Cham: Springer International Publishing; 2018. pp. 273-283

[41] Celikyurt U, Agacdiken A, Bozyel S, Argan O, Sade I, Vural A, et al. Assessment of shoulder pain and shoulder disability in patients with implantable cardioverter-defibrillator. Journal of Interventional Cardiac Electrophysiology. 2013;**36**(1):91-94

[42] Findikoglu G, Yildiz BS, Sanlialp M, Alihanoglu YI, Kilic ID, Evregul H, et al. Limitation of motion and

shoulder disabilities in patients with cardiac implantable electronic devices. International Journal of Rehabilitation Research. 2015;**38**(4):287-293

[43] Mahapatra S, Bybee KA, Bunch TJ, Espinosa RE, Sinak LJ, McGoon MD, et al. Incidence and predictors of cardiac perforation after permanent pacemaker placement. Heart Rhythm. 2005;**2**(9):907-911

[44] Cano O, Andres A, Alonso P, Osca J, Sancho-Tello MJ, Olague J, et al. Incidence and predictors of clinically relevant cardiac perforation associated with systematic implantation of active-fixation pacing and defibrillation leads: A single-Centre experience with over 3800 implanted leads. Europace. 2017;**19**(1):96-102

[45] Vanezis AP, Prasad R, Andrews R. Pacemaker leads and cardiac perforation. JRSM Open. 2017;**8**(3):2054270416681432

[46] Rajkumar CA, Claridge S, Jackson T, Behar J, Johnson J, Sohal M, et al. Diagnosis and management of iatrogenic cardiac perforation caused by pacemaker and defibrillator leads. Europace. 2017;**19**(6):1031-1037

[47] Barrett JF, Keat N. Artifacts in CT: Recognition and avoidance. Radiographics. 2004;**24**(6):1679-1691

[48] Merchant EE, Johnson SW, Nguyen P, Kang C, Mallon WK. Takotsubo cardiomyopathy: A case series and review of the literature. The Western Journal of Emergency Medicine. 2008;**9**(2):104-111

[49] Wei ZH, Dai Q, Wu H, Song J, Wang L, Xu B. Takotsubo cardiomyopathy after pacemaker implantation. Journal of Geriatric Cardiology. 2018;**15**(3):246-248

[50] Gardini A, Fracassi F, Boldi E, Albiero R. Apical ballooning syndrome

(takotsubo cardiomyopathy) after permanent dual-chamber pacemaker implantation. Case Reports in Cardiology. 2012;**2012**:308580

[51] Postema PG, Wiersma JJ, van der Bilt IA, Dekkers P, van Bergen PF. Takotsubo cardiomyopathy shortly following pacemaker implantation-case report and review of the literature. Netherlands Heart Journal. 2014;**22**(10):456-459

[52] Jefferies JL, Younis GA, Flamm SD, Rasekh A, Massumi A. Chest pain and diaphragmatic pacing after pacemaker implantation. Texas Heart Institute Journal. 2005;**32**(1):106-107

[53] Shah R, Qualls Z. Diaphragmatic stimulation caused by cardiac resynchronization treatment. CMAJ. 2016;**188**(10):E239

[54] Habib A, Lachman N, Christensen KN, Asirvatham SJ. The anatomy of the coronary sinus venous system for the cardiac electrophysiologist. Europace. 2009;**11**(Suppl 5):v15-v21

[55] Shah SS, Teague SD, Lu JC, Dorfman AL, Kazerooni EA, Agarwal PP. Imaging of the coronary sinus: Normal anatomy and congenital abnormalities. Radiographics. 2012;**32**(4):991-1008

[56] Moubarak G, Bouzeman A, Ollitrault J, Anselme F, Cazeau S. Phrenic nerve stimulation in cardiac resynchronization therapy. Journal of Interventional Cardiac Electrophysiology. 2014;**41**(1):15-21

[57] Banaszewski M, Stepinska J. Right heart perforation by pacemaker leads. Archives of Medical Science. 2012;**8**(1):11-13

[58] Namazi M, Karbasi-Afshar R, Safi M, Serati A. Diaphragmatic stimulation: A case of atrial lead

dislodgement and right atrium perforation. Indian Pacing and Electrophysiology Journal. 2008;**8**(2):133-136

[59] Tanabe K, Kotoda M, Nakashige D, Mitsui K, Ikemoto K, Matsukawa T. Sudden onset pacemaker-induced diaphragmatic twitching during general anesthesia. JA Clinical Reports. 2019;**5**(1):36

[60] Semmler V, Fichtner S, Lennerz C, Kolb C. Very late perforation of an implantable cardioverter defibrillator lead: A case report. The British Journal of General Practice. 2014;**64**(619):107-108

[61] Alla VM, Reddy YM, Abide W, Hee T, Hunter C. Delayed lead perforation: Can we ever let the guard down? Cardiology Research and Practice. 2010;**2010**:741-751. DOI: 10.4061/2010/741751

[62] Refaat MM, Hashash JG, Shalaby AA. Late perforation by cardiac implantable electronic device leads: Clinical presentation, diagnostic clues, and management. Clinical Cardiology. 2010;**33**(8):466-475

[63] Chao JA, Firstenberg MS. Delayed pacemaker lead perforations: Why unusual presentations should prompt an early multidisciplinary team approach. International Journal of Critical Illness and Injury Science. 2017;**7**(1):65-68

[64] Ibrahim M, Hasan R. Pacemaker-mediated angina. Experimental & Clinical Cardiology. 2013;**18**(1):35-37

[65] Duray GZ, Israel CW, Wegener FT, Hohnloser SH. Tachycardia after pacemaker implantation in a patient with complete atrioventricular block. Europace. 2007;**9**(10):900-903

[66] Mirescu NC, Muresan L, Farcas AD. A rare case of pacemaker induced tachycardia in an elderly woman with cor

triatriatum sinistrum. Oxford Medical Case Reports. 2017;**2017**(8):omx047

[67] Doppalapudi H. In: Ellenbogen KA, Wilkoff BL, Kay GN, Lau C, Auricchio A, editors. Timing Cycles of Implantable Devices. Philadelphia, PA: Elsevier; 2017. p. 961. DOI: 10.1016/B978-0-323-37804-8.00036-5

[68] Wessman DE, Stafford CM. The postcardiac injury syndrome: Case report and review of the literature. Southern Medical Journal. 2006;**99**(3):309-314

[69] Imazio M, Hoit BD. Post-cardiac injury syndromes: An emerging cause of pericardial diseases. International Journal of Cardiology. 2013;**168**(2):648-652

[70] Shvilkin A, Ellis ER, Gervino EV, Litvak AD, Buxton AE, Josephson ME. Painful left bundle branch block syndrome: Clinical and electrocardiographic features and further directions for evaluation and treatment. Heart Rhythm. 2016;**13**(1):226-232

[71] Ebrille E, DeSimone CV, Vaidya VR, Chahal AA, Nkomo VT, Asirvatham SJ. Ventricular pacing - electromechanical consequences and valvular function. Indian Pacing and Electrophysiology Journal. 2016;**16**(1):19-30

[72] Tops LF, Schalij MJ, Bax JJ. The effects of right ventricular apical pacing on ventricular function and dyssynchrony implications for therapy. Journal of the American College of Cardiology. 2009;**54**(9):764-776

[73] Virtanen KS, Heikkila J, Kala R, Siltanen P. Chest pain and rate-dependent left bundle branch block in patients with normal coronary arteriograms. Chest. 1982;**81**(3):326-331

[74] Sroubek J, Tugal D, Zimetbaum PJ, Shvilkin A, Buxton AE. Treatment

of painful left bundle branch
block syndrome with cardiac
resynchronization therapy or right-
ventricular pacing. HeartRhythm Case
Reports. 2019;**5**(6):321-324

[75] Mora B, Douard H, Barat JL,
Broustet JP. Simultaneous occurrence of
left heart block and chest pain during
exertion. Archives des maladies du coeur
et des vaisseaux. 1987;**80**(12):1807-1811

[76] Oladunjoye OO, Oladunjoye AO,
Oladiran O, Callans DJ, Schaller RD,
Licata A. Persistent exertional chest
pain in a marathon runner: Exercise-
induced, painful, left bundle branch
block syndrome treated with his-bundle
pacing. Mayo Clinic Proceedings:
Innovations, Quality & Outcomes.
2019;**3**(2):226-230

[77] Suryanarayana PG, Frankel DS,
Marchlinski FE, Schaller RD. Painful
left bundle branch block [corrected]
syndrome treated successfully
with permanent his bundle pacing.
HeartRhythm Case Reports.
2018;**4**(10):439-443

[78] Viles-Gonzalez JF, Mahata I,
Anter E, d'Avila A. Painful left bundle
branch block syndrome treated
with his bundle pacing. Journal of
Electrocardiology. 2018;**51**(6):1019-1022

Chapter 5

Aortic Dissection

Bina Nasim, Anas Mohammad, Sardar Zafar, Laji Mathew,
Ahmed Sajjad, Anis Shaikh and Ghulam Naroo

Abstract

Aortic dissection remains one of the rare but life-threatening causes of chest pain presenting to the emergency department. High index of suspicion is required for prompt diagnosis of the cases presenting to the ED. Symptoms may vary with extent and the progression of the dissection and may further complicate the diagnosis. Thus, patients may present with features of acute MI, CVA, or other end-organ ischemia. Hypertension at presentation may be an important clue for diagnosis of underlying dissection. In low risk patients, D dimer may become a useful screening tool. In patients with high index of suspicion, the choice of investigation will depend on the overall stability of the patient and extent of end-organ ischemia. Stable patients may benefit from CT angiography due to its widespread availability and speed of acquisition. Diagnosis may be challenging for hemodynamically unstable patients in centers where the resources are limited. Transesophageal echocardiography may provide diagnosis in such patients at bedside or in the emergency department. Prompt investigations are required to accurately define the type and extent of damage so that the patient receives life-saving measures in a timely manner.

Keywords: aortic dissection, D dimer, CT angiography, transesophageal echocardiography

1. Classification

Aortic dissection (AD) has been conventionally classified based on anatomical considerations (**Figure 1**).

1.1 Anatomical classification

1.1.1 DeBakey classification

This classification takes into consideration the site of origin of the intimal tear and classifies AD into three types:

- Type I—Originating in the ascending aorta and propagating at least to the aortic arch.

- Type II—Originating and confined to the ascending aorta.

- Type III—Originating in the descending aorta.

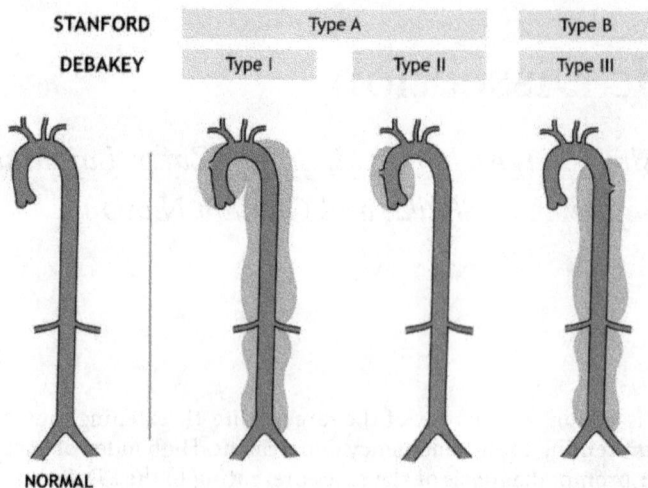

Figure 1.
Anatomical classification of aortic dissection.

1.1.2 Stanford classification

This classification takes into consideration involvement of the ascending aorta irrespective of the origin of the intimal tear:

• Type A—Dissection involves the ascending aorta.

• Type B—Dissection spares the ascending aorta.

Stanford classification is widely used to drive further decision-making and management as any involvement of the ascending aorta (type A) is a surgical emergency, whereas type B can be managed conservatively.

1.2 Etiological classification

Aortic dissection can also be classified based on etiological considerations.

1.2.1 Sporadic

Not associated with any known congenital or genetically mediated syndromes.

1.2.2 Genetically mediated

Associated with known genetic syndromes like Marfan's syndrome, Ehlers-Danlos syndrome, Turner syndrome, and Loeys-Dietz syndrome.

1.2.3 Congenital cardiovascular defects

Bicuspid aortic valve, coarctation of aorta, and annuloaortic ectasia.

1.2.4 Traumatic

Prior cardiac surgery, blunt injury, and cardiac catheterization.

1.3 Newer classification

With advancement of treatment approach in cases previously managed conservatively, especially with endovascular interventions, recent classifications have taken into consideration other factors like, the duration of symptom onset, evolution of complications, and extent of involved segments.

1.3.1 Dissect classification

The DISSECT classification system is a mnemonic-based approach with relevance to the therapeutic considerations, including endovascular management. The six features of aortic dissection include duration of disease, intimal tear location, size of the dissected aorta, segmental extent of aortic involvement, clinical complications of the dissection, and thrombus within the aortic false lumen [1].

1.3.2 Penn ABC classification

The Penn ABC classification further divides type A aortic dissection based on evolution of complications:

- Aa—Absence of branch vessel malperfusion or circulatory collapse

- Ab—Branch vessel malperfusion with ischemia

- Ac—Circulatory collapse with or without cardiac involvement

- Abc—Both branch vessel malperfusion and circulatory collapse (localized and generalized ischemia)

1.3.3 Classification based on duration of symptoms

More recently type B aortic dissection has been classified based on duration of symptom onset [2]:

- Acute—less than 2 weeks

- Subacute—2 weeks to 92 days

- Chronic—>92 days

2. Pathophysiology

The pathophysiology of AD involves the breakdown of the intima and/or the media. The initiating event is an intimal tear. Less commonly rupture of the vasa vasorum may be the initiating event. Initial tear is commonly at the site of greatest hydraulic stress which are the right lateral wall of the ascending aorta in about 50–65% of the cases and the proximal segment of the descending aorta (20–30%) [3]. Subsequently, intramural extension of the bleeding both longitudinally and circumferentially causes the separation of aortic wall layers creating a true lumen and a false lumen. A further intimal tear may create a communication between the false lumen and true lumen. The dissection can extend in antegrade or retrograde

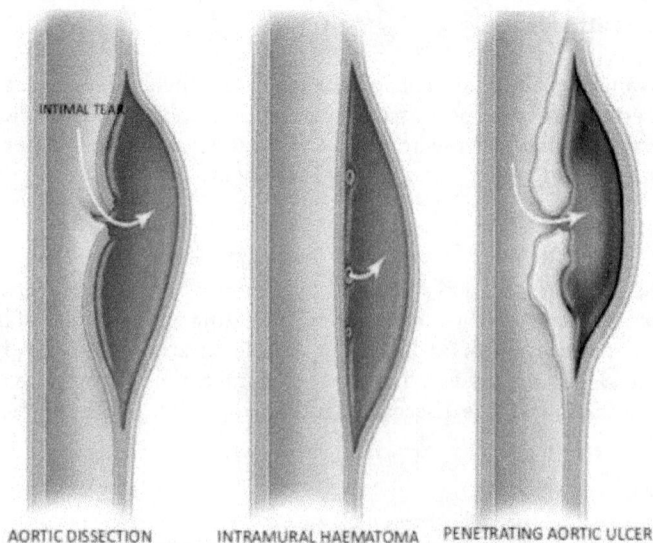

AORTIC DISSECTION   INTRAMURAL HAEMATOMA   PENETRATING AORTIC ULCER

Figure 2.
Acute aortic syndrome.

directions from the site of origin leading to complications including acute aortic insufficiency, cardiac tamponade, and organ ischemia and with disruption of the adventitial layer may lead to aortic rupture.

Intramural hematoma (IMH) is characterized by bleeding confined to the medial layer with no intimal tear visualized by current imaging studies.

Rarely ulceration of an atherosclerotic lesion penetrating to the medial layer may give rise to a penetrating aortic ulcer with similar consequences as of AD.

These three conditions, namely, AD, IMH, and penetrating aortic ulcer, are categorized under the broader category of acute aortic syndrome (AAS) (**Figure 2**) [4].

3. Predisposing conditions

Factors that increase the risk of aortic dissection in a person's life include the following;

3.1 Age and sex

Aortic dissection tends to occur more in men between 60 and 80 years old, whereas women are generally older than men having aortic dissection [5]. However both men and women can develop these conditions at any age, but in females the outcome is worse. On the other hand, familial aortic dissections occur in younger patients as compared to sporadic aortic dissection [6].

3.2 Hypertension

Systemic hypertension is the most important predisposing condition for aortic dissection. It could be either an acute, transient, abrupt rise in blood pressure leading to aortic dissection by various mechanisms like strenuous resistance exercises, weight lifting or illicit use of drugs like cocaine, egotism, and energy drink usage [7, 8]. While chronic or long-term hypertension keeps greater pressure on atherosclerotic arterial walls, leading to intimal tear and aortic aneurysm.

3.3 Genetic disorders

People having specific genetic conditions have a higher incidence of aortic dissection, like Marfan's syndrome, Turners syndrome, Ehlers-Danlos syndrome, annuloaortic ectasia, adult polycystic kidney disease, Noonan syndrome, and osteogenesis imperfecta. Mostly patients with Marfan's syndrome who develop aortic dissection are young, around 40 years old, and have family history of Marfan's syndrome and aortic dissection [9].

3.4 Bicuspid aortic valve

Bicuspid aortic valve usually leads to aortic dissection of ascending aorta, because of severe loss of elastic fibers in the media wall. Patients with bicuspid valves associated with aortic dissection are younger below 40 years age [10].

3.5 Coarctation of aorta

The most common area for congenital coarctation of aorta is the site of ductus arteriosus, where the aorta is focally narrowed. That area is usually underdeveloped, hypoplastic, and small, affecting the layers of the aorta, and increases the risk for aortic dissection.

3.6 Inflammatory or infectious conditions

Inflammatory or infectious diseases that lead to vasculitis (like giant cell arteritis, rheumatoid arthritis, takayasu arteritis, syphilitic aortitis, etc.) affect the vaso vasorum or small arteries that supply blood to the aortic wall [11]. When these small arteries are compromised, they lead to the ischemic injury to the aortic wall and predisposes to aortic dissection. For example, in tertiary syphilis, inflammation begins at adventitia of the aortic arch leading to obliterative endarteritis of the vasa vasorum, luminal narrowing, ischemic injury of medial aortic arch, and finally loss of elastic support and vessel dilatation.

3.7 Blunt chest trauma

The aortic area most commonly involved in blunt chest trauma is the proximal descending aorta, due to its relative mobility over fixed abdominal aorta which is held in place by ligamentum arteriosum. Usually an acute deceleration injury in motor vehicle accident leads to aortic rupture or dissection.

3.8 Aortic instrumentation or previous heart surgery

Cardiac surgery or instrumentation for coronary or valvular heart diseases can be complicated by aortic tear, abnormal dilatation of aorta, and risk for aortic dissection [12].

3.9 Pregnancy and delivery

Both pregnancy and delivery are independent risk factors for aortic dissection [13], but with the presence of other connective tissue diseases like Marfan's syndrome or bicuspid aortic valve, the risk usually multiplies. In pregnancy, aortic dissection occurs most commonly in third trimester due to hyper dynamic metabolic state and hormonal effects on the vasculature.

3.10 Fluoroquinolone usage

Some observational studies relate an increased association of aortic dissection or aneurysm with fluoroquinolone usage [14].

4. Clinical features of aortic dissection

The signs and symptoms of aortic dissection depends upon the extent of dissection and compression of adjacent vascular structures.

4.1 Symptoms

4.1.1 Chest pain

The most common symptom is severe pain of sudden onset, described by patient as sharp stabbing or tearing type. When pain localized to anterior chest wall, neck, or jaw, the point of origin of the aortic dissection is from the ascending aorta, and when it is localized to the interscapular area, abdomen, and back, the descending aorta is usually involved.

Pain that is localized to the abdomen must raise the possibility of involvement of the mesenteric artery.

In few cases the patient may present with pleuritic pain if pericardial hemorrhage occurs.

Dissection may present rarely without pain only and mostly in older patients in cases that involve the ascending aorta. Such patients also have more instances of stroke, heart failure, and syncope.

4.1.2 Syncope

Usually happens in aortic dissection presenting with cardiac tamponade or brachiocephalic vessel involvement and occurs in up to 10% of patients.

4.2 Signs

4.2.1 Hypertension

Seen in 30% of type A and 70% of type B disease.

4.2.2 Hypotension

Seen with ascending aortic dissection and may be due to aortic rupture leading to carotid tamponade (more in females), acute aortic regurgitation, acute MI, hemothorax ,or hemoperitoneum.

4.2.3 Transient pulse deficits

This results from the intimal flap or hematoma blocking or compressing the artery. It is common in dissection involving the aortic arch and thoracic and abdominal aorta.

Patients who presented with pulse deficits had more chances of having hypotension, coma, or neurological deficits. Such patients also had higher rates of complications and mortality.

4.2.4 Cardiac murmurs

Aortic dissection involving the aortic valve results in aortic regurgitation and an early diastolic murmur in the Erb's point (Austin Flint murmur). It occurs in about 50–75% of all ascending aortic dissections.

4.2.5 Focal neurological deficits

Occurs when the aortic dissection involves the proximal branch arteries and compression of adjacent structures. The deficits may be:

- Stroke/altered consciousness

- Horner Syndrome (compression of cervical sympathetic ganglia)

- Hoarseness of voice (compression of the left recurrent laryngeal nerve)

- Acute paraplegic (spinal cord ischemia from intercostal vessel compression)

Also seen are:

- Collapsing pulse

- Wide pulse pressure

- Congestive cardiac failure

- Pleural effusion (commonly left-sided)

- Pulsating neck swelling

5. Work-up/diagnosis

In chronological order as the patient is admitted into ER with a clinical picture suggestive of aortic dissection:

5.1 Electrocardiography

ECG changes may mimic acute cardiac ischemia, which make it further difficult to distinguish aortic dissection from acute myocardial infarction in the presence of chest pain.

If the dissection involves the coronary ostia, the right coronary artery can be affected, which will lead to ST segment elevation in a similar pattern to inferior wall infarction.

In most cases, there will be non-specific ECG changes, or ECG can be normal.

5.2 Blood investigations

CBC: there may be **leukocytosis** due to stress state. **Low hemoglobin** and hematocrit suggests bleeding (dissection is leaking or has ruptured).

Elevated creatinine and BUN may indicate involvement of renal arteries (in such scenario you would expect hematuria, oliguria, or anuria), or it may indicate dehydration due to pre-renal blood loss (dissection is leaking or has ruptured).

Troponin I and T may be elevated if the dissection has involved the coronary arteries and caused myocardial ischemia.

LDH (lactate dehydrogenase) may be elevated due to hemolysis in the false lumen.

D dimer: high negative predictive value. **Aortic dissection is less likely if D dimer is negative** [15].

5.3 Chest radiography

Widening of mediastinum is the classic finding (approximately 60% of cases), but it may not reveal any abnormality. In any case it should not delay the performance of further imaging as CT or MRI [16]. A tortuous aorta (common in hypertensive patients) may be mistaken for widened mediastinum; other differential diagnoses for widened mediastinum include enlarged thyroid, lymphoma, tumors, and adenopathy [17].

Hemothorax is expected to be seen as blood can accumulate in pleural space following dissection rupture.

Ring sign (aortic displacement more than 5 mm past the calcific aortic intima) and abnormal aortic contour can be seen in some patients.

Other radiological abnormalities can be seen including esophageal deviation, tracheal deviation to the right, depression of left mediastinal bronchus, left apical cap, pleural effusion, and loss of paratracheal stripe.

5.4 Echocardiography

Transesophageal echocardiography has higher diagnostic index (sensitivity 99% and specificity 97%) than transthoracic echocardiography (sensitivity 80% and specificity 90%) [18].

TEE is as accurate as CT and MRI, and it can be used at bedside which makes it suitable for hemodynamically unstable patients.

Limitations of transesophageal echocardiography:

- Operator dependent.

- Difficulty in obese patients.

- Not suitable for patients with esophageal stenosis or varicosities.

- Narrow intercostal space, pulmonary emphysema, and mechanical ventilation decrease its accuracy.

- Upper ascending aorta and arch may not be evaluated well.

- False-positive results may occur due to reverberations in the ascending aorta [19].

5.5 Computed tomography

CT with contrast is used more frequently in emergency department settings, only on hemodynamically stable patients who do not have adverse reaction to the intravenous contrast agents.

A 2014 guideline form American College of Radiology recommends CT angiography as the definite modality if there is high clinical suspicion for aortic dissection [16].

CTA provides detailed anatomic definition of the dissection and information about plaque formation.

Spiral (helical) CT is associated with higher rate of detection and better resolution than incremental CT scanning. Imaging information, including type of the lesion, location of pathologic lesion, extent of the disease, and evaluation of the true and false lumen can be assessed quickly and help the surgeon plan the operation [16, 20].

Limitations of CT:

- Cannot provide information about aortic regurgitation.

- CTA not suitable for patient with renal impairment or allergy to contrast material.

- Hemodynamic unstable patients cannot be shifted to radiology department.

5.6 Smooth-muscle myosin heavy-chain assay

Performed in the first 24 hours. **Levels are higher in the first 3 hours**; a 2.5-fold increase has a sensitivity of 91% and specificity of 98% for aortic dissection.

5.7 Measurement of the degradation products of plasma fibrin and fibrinogen

Plasma fibrin degradation product level (FDP) of **12.6 μg/mL or higher** is suggestive of the possibility of aortic dissection with false lumen in symptomatic patient.

Plasma fibrin degradation product level (FDP) of 5.6 μg/mL or higher is suggestive of the possibility of dissection with complete thrombosis of the false lumen [21].

5.8 Magnetic resonance imaging (MRI)

MRI has 98% sensitivity and specificity in detection of thoracic aortic dissection.

MRI shows the site on intimal tear, type and extent of dissection, presence of aortic insufficiency, as well as surrounding mediastinal structures. It has the advantage of not using contrast material; thus, it is preferred in patients with renal impairment or allergic to iodine [22].

Limitations of MRI:

- Not suitable for hemodynamically unstable patients.

- Requires much more time than CT.

- Not suitable for patients with pacemaker and other metallic implants [23].

5.9 Aortography

5.9.1 The gold-standard diagnostic modality for aortic dissection

Benefits include accurate visualization of the true and false lumen, intimal flap, aortic regurgitation, and coronary arteries.

Limits of aortography:

- Invasive procedure.

- Not suitable for patient with renal impairment or allergic to contrast.

- Not suitable for hemodynamically unstable patients.

- The false lumen and intimal flap may not be visualized if the false channel is thrombosed.

- Simultaneous opacification of the true and false lumen may mask the dissection.

5.9.2 Diagnosis

Diagnosis is usually done through imaging. The choice of the imaging technique depends on the patient condition (whether he is hemodynamically stable or not).

Chest radiography is the initial basic imaging technique, but it may reveal no abnormality.

Further imaging options like computed tomography (CT) and CT angiography with three-dimensional reconstruction are of higher diagnostic value.

Magnetic resonance imaging (MRI) is as accurate as CT and may benefit patients who have adverse reaction to intravenous drug agents.

In hemodynamically unstable patient, echocardiography is ideal.

Aortography is the gold-standard diagnostic modality.

6. Differential diagnosis

6.1 Myocardial infarction

Typically presents with severe substernal or left-sided chest discomfort radiating to shoulders or left arm and shortness of breath and can be differentiated from AD by the typical ECG changes and the rise in the cardiac markers.

6.2 Myocarditis

Viral myocarditis is often preceded by flu-like symptoms, fever, joint pain, or features of upper respiratory tract infection. These patients usually present with heart failure, and ECHO is done to exclude it from other causes of heart failure.

6.3 Pericarditis or cardiac tamponade

Presents with sharp chest pain and may have a pericardial friction rub. Patients with tamponade present with cardiogenic shock and have low-voltage ECG with electrical alternans and enlarged cardiac shadow on the Chest X-ray.

6.4 Pulmonary embolism

Classically presents with sudden onset of chest pain, shortness of breath, and hypoxia. In patients suspected to have pulmonary embolism, CT pulmonary angiogram is the definitive investigation to establish the diagnosis.

6.5 Tension pneumothorax

Patients present with sudden onset of sharp chest pain and desaturation with absent breath sounds. Diagnosis can be established by Chest X-ray.

6.6 Esophageal rupture

Often preceded by history of forceful vomiting, upper gastrointestinal endoscopy or instrumentation. Chest X-ray shows pneumomediastinum, pneumothorax, or pleural effusion.

7. Management of aortic dissection

7.1 Acute management of aortic dissection involves immediate resuscitation

- Intensive blood pressure monitoring preferably with arterial line to maintain SBP between 100 and 120 mmHg and heart rate < 60/min, to prevent the dissection from expanding. This lowering of blood pressure can be attained with:

  ○ First line—Beta-blockade using labetalol (20 mg iv initially, followed by either 20–80 mg iv boluses every 10 min to a maximal dose of 300 mg or an infusion of 0.5–2 mg/min IV), esmolol (250–500 mcg/kg IV loading dose; then infuse at 25–50 mcg/kg/min, and titrate to maximum dose of 300 mcg/kg/min).

  ○ Second line—In patients with asthma, allergy, or any contraindication to beta-blockade, calcium channel blockers diltiazem and verapamil can be used.

  ○ Third line—Vasodilator therapy. If blood pressure remains above 120mmHg and heart rate < 60/min, nitroprusside infusion (0.25–0.5 mcg/kg/min titrated to a maximum of 10 mcg/kg/min) can be initiated. This vasodilator therapy should not be used without first lowering heart rate with beta-/calcium channel blocker.

  ○ Pain control using iv opioids (tramadol, morphine, fentanyl)

  ○ Specific management depends on site of dissection

7.1.1 Acute type A dissection

Acute type A dissection is a surgical emergency with a mortality of 1–2% per hour, as these patients are at high risk of complications such as aortic regurgitation, tamponade, myocardial infarction due to compression of the coronary ostium, stroke, and aortic rupture [24].

This excludes patients with significant comorbidities including prior debilitating stroke, ischemic heart disease, renal failure, malignancy, advancing age, and hemorrhagic stroke, which are associated with a bad prognosis.

These patients should also be assessed for any underlying coronary artery disease or any aortic valve disease by intraoperative transesophageal ECHO to identify any wall motion abnormality or aortic valvular defect.

In the International Registry of Aortic Dissection (IRAD) review of 547 patients in which 80 percent of type A patients were treated surgically and the remaining 20 percent were treatment medically, inpatient mortality rates were 27 and 56 percent for surgical and medically treated patients. Medically treated patients were those with advanced comorbidities and aged individuals with poor prognosis [25].

Poor prognostic factors predicting increased mortality in type A patients according to the IRAD study included advanced age, tamponade at presentation, prior myocardial infarction, prior stroke, ischemia involving kidney or other viscera, advance renal or lung disease, and previous aortic valve replacement [25–31].

Open surgical repair for type A patients involves resection of the dissecting aneurysm and removal of intimal tear, closure of false lumen and repair of aorta using synthetic graft, and aortic valve repair/replacement. Repair of the aortic arch may also be needed depending on the extent of the pathology.

Patients with genetic disease like Marfan causing Aortic regurgitation, bicuspid aortic valve or aortitis need aortic valve replacement [32].

An alternative to open surgical repair in type A patients with ischemic complications like renal, mesenteric, and peripheral ischemia is endovascular stent grafting.

A novel approach involves the hybrid repair of type A dissection with "frozen elephant trunk repair technique," which involves open surgical repair of the ascending aorta in the form of a traditional elephant trunk and endoscopic stent grafting to repair the descending aorta.

Studies have compared the total arch replacement using the frozen elephant trunk repair technique (FET) with the hemi-arch replacement (AHR) for the type A ascending aortic dissection in which the survival for the patients after 5 years was 95.3% for the FET group and 69.0% for the AHR group, indicating that FET techniques prevent further operations for the complications because of the false lumen [25, 33–35].

7.1.2 Type B aortic dissection

Medical management is preferred for uncomplicated cases of type B aortic dissections unless the dissection or aneurysm expands, ischemic complications or aortic rupture occurs, or the patient has persistent uncontrolled hypertension or chest pain, when surgical treatment or endovascular grafting is to be considered.

Conservative treatment for type B patients involves optimal BP control and long-term surveillance with imaging.

In the IRAD study of 384 patients with type B aortic dissection [36], 73 percent of patients were treated medically with mortality rate of 13% within the first week of admission. Factors associated with increased mortality were shock on presentation, widened mediastinum, excessively dilated aorta ($\geq$6 cm), periaortic hematoma, patients with coma or altered consciousness, mesenteric or limb ischemia, acute renal failure, and patients who were treated surgically.

Endovascular stent grafting is done with the stent covering the dissection leading to thrombosis causing closure of false lumen.

Open surgical repair is rarely done in type B patients. It may be needed in those patients with genetic condition like Marfan's syndrome in whom endovascular repair is difficult.

Several trials have compared medical management with endovascular stent grafting in uncomplicated patients with type B aortic dissection demonstrating that at 2 years there is no difference in survival in either of the endovascular versus medical groups (89% versus 96%) [37]; however at 5 years the occurrence of the aortic complications is reduced in the endovascular group improving late outcome [38].

7.2 Long-term management

Optimal blood pressure control is needed to prevent recurrence or aneurysm formation. This is best achieved by oral combination antihypertensive therapy often including oral beta-blockers. Target blood pressure of less than 120/80 mmHg is preferred.

Screening of first-degree relatives should be performed with transthoracic ECHO (TTE) to look for aortic aneurysm.

At discharge transesophageal ECHO (TEE), magnetic resonance imaging (MRA), or CT angiography should be performed to detect for any leak, and serial images should be done at 3, 6, and 12 months to look for any recurrence, expansion, aneurysmal formation, or leak. MRA is preferred to TEE as is it noninvasive. In patients with renal impairment, MRI can be done without gadolinium.

8. Prognosis

8.1 Type a aortic dissection patients

Untreated patients with type A dissections have a mortality rate of 1–2% per hour because of its association with high risk of complications of aortic rupture, tamponade, aortic regurgitation, ischemic complications of myocardial infarction, and stroke [24].

According to the IRAD follow-up study of 303 patients with type A dissection who were discharged from the hospital, surgically treated patients were 273 (90.1%), and medically treated patients were 30 (9.9%). Surgically treated patients had a 1-year survival of 96.1 ± 2.4% and 3-year survival of 90.5 + 3.9%, whereas the medically treated type A dissection patients had a 1-year survival of 88.6 + 12.2% and 3-year survival of 68.7 + 19.8% [39].

8.2 Type B aortic dissection

Uncomplicated type B patients have an overall survival rate of 90% with immediate medical management with effective control of blood pressure [36].

However in type B patients with complications of aortic rupture, expansion of dissection or ischemic complications of organ hypoperfusion the mortality rates were high. According to the IRAD study, the overall inhospital mortality rate was 13% during the first week, for all type B aortic dissection patients. Mortality rate in type B dissection patients with complications, undergoing surgical management, was 32.1%, whereas in those treated with medical management alone, the mortality rate was 9.6% and was 6.5% for those treated with endovascular approach [36].

The 3-year survival rate for type B patients who were discharged from the hospital according to the IRAD registry was 77.6 ± 6.6% for medically treated patients, 82.8 ± 18.9% for surgically treated patients, and 76.2 ± 25.2% for those treated with endovascular approach [40].

Author details

Bina Nasim, Anas Mohammad, Sardar Zafar, Laji Mathew, Ahmed Sajjad, Anis Shaikh and Ghulam Naroo*
Rashid Hospital, Dubai, United Arab Emirates

*Address all correspondence to: gynaroo@dha.gov.ae

IntechOpen

References

[1] Dake MD et al. DISSECT: A new mnemonic-based approach to the categorization of aortic dissection. European Journal of Vascular and Endovascular Surgery. 2013;**46**(2):175-190

[2] Mid-term outcomes and aortic remodeling after thoracic endovascular repair for acute, subacute, and chronic aortic dissection: The VIRTUE registry. European Journal of Vascular and Endovascular Surgery. 2014;**48**(4):363-371

[3] Hagan PG, Nienaber CA, Isselbacher EM, et al. The international registry of acute aortic dissection (IRAD): New insights into an old disease. JAMA. 2000;**383**:897

[4] Vilacosta I, San Roman JA. Acute aortic syndrome. Heart. 2001;**85**:365-368

[5] Fattori R, Nienaber CA, Mehta RH, Richartz BM, Evangelista A, Petzsch M, et al. Gender-related differences in acute aortic dissection. International registry of acute aortic dissection. Circulation. 2004;**109**(24):3014

[6] Chou AS, Ma WG, Mok SC, Ziganshin BA, Peterss S, et al. Do familial aortic dissections tend to occur at the same age? The Annals of Thoracic Surgery. 2017;**103**(2):546. Epub 2016 Aug 25

[7] Spittell PC, Spittell JA Jr, Joyce JW, Tajik AJ, et al. Clinical features and differential diagnosis of aortic dissection: Experience with 236 cases (1980 through 1990). Mayo Clinic Proceedings. 1993;**68**(7):642

[8] Howard DP, Banerjee A, Fairhead JF, Perkins J, et al. Population-based study of incidence and outcome of acute aortic dissection and premorbid risk factor control: 10-year results from the Oxford vascular study. Circulation. 2013;**127**(20):2031

[9] Januzzi JL, Isselbacher EM, Fattori R, et al. Characterizing the young patient with aortic dissection: Results from the international registry of aortic dissection (IRAD), international registry of aortic dissection (IRAD). Journal of the American College of Cardiology. 2004;**43**(4):665

[10] Nistri S, Sorbo MD, Marin M, Palisi M, Scognamiglio R, et al. Aortic root dilatation in young men with normally functioning bicuspid aortic valves. Heart. 1999;**82**(1):19

[11] Barison A, Nugara C, Barletta V, Todiere G, et al. Asymptomatic Takayasu aortitis complicated by type B dissection. Circulation. 2015;**132**(22):e254-e255

[12] Bautista D, Nunez-Gil U, Cerrato E, Salinas P, Varbella F, et al. Incidence, management, and immediate- and long-term outcomes after iatrogenic aortic dissection during diagnostic or interventional coronary procedures, registry on aortic iatrogenic dissection (RAID) investigators. Circulation. 2015;**131**(24):2114. Pub 2015 Apr 17

[13] Roman MJ, Pugh NL, Hendershot TP, Devereux RB, et al. Aortic complications associated with pregnancy in Marfan syndrome: The NHLBI national registry of genetically triggered thoracic aortic aneurysms and cardiovascular conditions. Journal of the American Heart Association. 2016;**5**(8):e004052. Pub 2016 Aug 11

[14] Lee CC, Lee MG, Hsieh R, Porta L, et al. Oral fluoroquinolone and the risk of aortic dissection. Journal of the American College of Cardiology. 2018;**72**(12):1369

[15] Suzuki T, Distante A, Zizza A, Trimarchi S, Villani M, Salerno

Uriarte JA, et al. Diagnosis of acute aortic dissection by D-dimer: The international registry of acute aortic dissection substudy on biomarkers (IRAD-bio) experience. Circulation. 2009;**119**(20):2702-2707

[16] Latson LA Jr, Jacobs JE, Abbara S, et al, Expert Panels on Cardiac Imaging. ACR appropriateness criteria® acute chest pain - suspected aortic dissection. American college of radiology. 2014. 11 p. [Accessed: 28 November 2018]

[17] Hagan PG, Nienaber CA, Isselbacher EM, Bruckman D, Karavite DJ, Russman PL, et al. The international registry of acute aortic dissection (IRAD): New insights into an old disease. Journal of the American Medical Association. 2000;**283**(7):897-903

[18] Meredith EL, Masani ND. Echocardiography in the emergency assessment of acute aortic syndromes. European Journal of Echocardiography. 2009;**10**(1):i31-i39

[19] Adachi H, Kyo S, Takamoto S, Kimura S, Yokote Y, Omoto R. Early diagnosis and surgical intervention of acute aortic dissection by transesophageal color flow mapping. Circulation. 1990;**82**(5 Suppl): IV19-IV23

[20] Cigarroa JE, Isselbacher EM, DeSanctis RW, Eagle KA. Diagnostic imaging in the evaluation of suspected aortic dissection. Old standards and new directions. The New England Journal of Medicine. 1993;**328**(1):35-43

[21] Hagiwara A, Shimbo T, Kimira A, Sasaki R, Kobayashi K, Sato T. Using fibrin degradation products level to facilitate diagnostic evaluation of potential acute aortic dissection. Journal of Thrombosis and Thrombolysis. 2013;**35**(1):15-22

[22] Nienaber CA, von Kodolitsch Y, Nicolas V, Siglow V, Piepho A,

Brockhoff C, et al. The diagnosis of thoracic aortic dissection by noninvasive imaging procedures. The New England Journal of Medicine. 1993;**328**(1):1-9

[23] Nienaber CA, Spielmann RP, von Kodolitsch Y, Siglow V, Piepho A, Jaup T, et al. Diagnosis of thoracic aortic dissection. Magnetic resonance imaging versus transesophageal echocardiography. Circulation. 1992;**85**(2):434-447

[24] Nienaber CA, Eagle KA. Aortic dissection: New frontiers in diagnosis and management: Part I: From etiology to diagnostic strategies. Circulation. 2003;**108**:628

[25] Mehta RH, Suzuki T, Hagan PG, et al. Predicting death in patients with acute type a aortic dissection. Circulation. 2002;**105**:200

[26] Miller DC, Mitchell RS, Oyer PE, et al. Independent determinants of operative mortality for patients with aortic dissections. Circulation. 1984;**70**:I153

[27] Haverich A, Miller DC, Scott WC, et al. Acute and chronic aortic dissections--determinants of long-term outcome for operative survivors. Circulation. 1985;**72**:II22

[28] Pansini S, Gagliardotto PV, Pompei E, et al. Early and late risk factors in surgical treatment of acute type a aortic dissection. The Annals of Thoracic Surgery. 1998;**66**:779

[29] Kawahito K, Adachi H, Yamaguchi A, Ino T. Preoperative risk factors for hospital mortality in acute type a aortic dissection. The Annals of Thoracic Surgery. 2001;**71**:1239

[30] Chiappini B, Schepens M, Tan E, et al. Early and late outcomes of acute type a aortic dissection: Analysis of risk factors in 487 consecutive patients. European Heart Journal. 2005;**26**:180

[31] Mehta RH, O'Gara PT, Bossone E, et al. Acute type a aortic dissection in the elderly: Clinical characteristics, management, and outcomes in the current era. Journal of the American College of Cardiology. 2002;**40**:685

[32] DeSanctis RW, Doroghazi RM, AustenWG,BuckleyMJ.Aorticdissection. The New England Journal of Medicine. 1987;**317**:1060

[33] Murzi M, Tiwari KK, Farneti PA, Glauber M. Might type a acute dissection repair with the addition of a frozen elephant trunk improve long-term survival compared to standard repair? Interactive Cardiovascular and Thoracic Surgery. 2010;**11**:98

[34] Uchida N, Katayama A, Tamura K, et al. Long-term results of the frozen elephant trunk technique for extended aortic arch disease. European Journal of Cardio-Thoracic Surgery. 2010;**37**:1338

[35] Uchida N, Shibamura H, Katayama A, et al. Operative strategy for acute type a aortic dissection: Ascending aortic or hemiarch versus total arch replacement with frozen elephant trunk. The Annals of Thoracic Surgery. 2009;**87**:773

[36] Suzuki T, Mehta RH, Ince H, et al. Clinical profiles and outcomes of acute type B aortic dissection in the current era: Lessons from the international registry of aortic dissection (IRAD). Circulation. 2003;**108**(Suppl. 1):II312

[37] Nienaber CA, Rousseau H, Eggebrecht H, et al. Randomized comparison of strategies for type B aortic dissection: The INvestigation of STEnt grafts in aortic dissection (INSTEAD) trial. Circulation. 2009;**120**:2519

[38] Nienaber CA, Kische S, Rousseau H, et al. Endovascular repair of type B aortic dissection: Long-term results of the randomized investigation of stent grafts in aortic dissection trial. Circulation. Cardiovascular Interventions. 2013;**6**:407.40

[39] Tsai TT, Evangelista A, Nienaber CA, Trimarchi S, Sechtem U, Fattori R, et al. Long-Term Survival in Patients Presenting with Type a Acute Aortic Dissection: Insights from the International Registry of Acute Aortic Dissection (IRAD) Circulation. Vol. 114. 2006. pp. I350-I356

[40] Tsai TT, Fattori R, Trimarchi S, Isselbacher E, Myrmel T, Evangelista A, et al. Long-term survival in patients presenting with type b acute aortic dissection. Insights from the international registry of Acute Aortic Dissection. Circulation. July 2006;**114** (1 suppl):1350-1356

Chapter 6

Takotsubo Syndrome and Nitric Oxide Bioavailability

Michael Demosthenous, Konstantinos Triantafyllou
and Nikolaos Koumallos

Abstract

Takotsubo cardiomyopathy, also known as broken heart syndrome or stress cardiomyopathy, is a form of transient left ventricular dysfunction. Severe apical and mid left ventricular hypokinesis with hypercontractility of the basal segments is observed. Numerous underlying causes and pathophysiological mechanisms have been proposed including sudden sympathetic activation and increase in the circulating levels of catecholamines resulting in multivessel coronary spasm. Another possible mechanism related to catecholamine-mediated myocardial stunning is direct myocyte injury. Increasing data show that endothelial dysfunction and depleted nitric oxide bioavailability are common in patients with Takotsubo cardiomyopathy. In this chapter we examine in depth the relation between endothelial dysfunction and Takotsubo syndrome.

Keywords: Takotsubo cardiomyopathy, broken heart syndrome, nitric oxide, endothelial dysfunction, ADMA

1. Introduction

Takotsubo cardiomyopathy (TC), also known as broken heart syndrome or stress cardiomyopathy, is a form of transient left ventricular (LV) dysfunction. Severe apical and mid left ventricular hypokinesis with hypercontractility of the basal segments is observed [1–4]. The name derives from the fact that the shape of the LV of patients with Takotsubo syndrome resembles the octopus fishing pot used in Japan where the first studied case of TC was done by Sato et al. in the early 1990s (**Figure 1(a)** and **(b)**).

The InterTAK diagnostic score is a score that predicts the probability of Takotsubo cardiomyopathy and differentiates form acute coronary syndrome. Female sex and emotional stress yield the highest score. Other predisposing factors include physical stress, psychiatric disorders, and neurological disorders.

Takotsubo cardiomyopathy usually presents with shortness of breath, hypotension, angina or syncope. Laboratory work may reveal elevated troponin levels. Electrocardiogram may show signs of ischemia, such as T wave inversion or even ST elevation [1]. Coronary angiogram typically reveals normal coronary arteries.

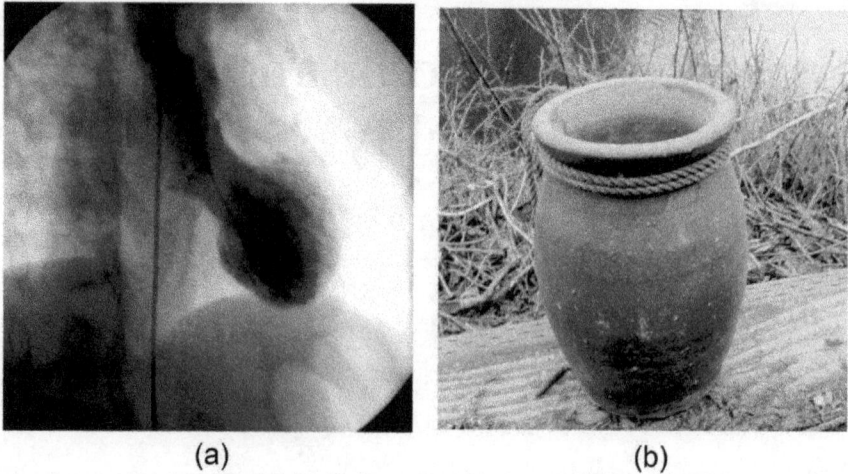

Figure 1.
(a) Angiogram of a patient with Takotsubo cardiomyopathy showing the apical balloning of the left ventricle. (b) The Takotsubo fishing pot after syndrome was named. You can appreciate the resemblance with angiographic image on the left.

2. Pathophysiology

The pathophysiology of TC is quite complex and a number of different mechanisms have been proposed, including sudden sympathetic activation and increase in the circulating levels of catecholamines resulting in multivessel coronary spasm [5–15]. Coronary vasospasm and sympathetic mediated microvascular dysfunction have been observed in patients with TC.

According to Gupta et al. [16], the pathophysiology of sympathetic mediated coronary vasospasm and microvascular dysfunction can be divided in two phases.

According to the authors, the first phase starts with cognitive centers of the brain. As a response to stress, the hypothalamic-pituitary-adrenal axis is activated and releases catecholamines. In the case of TC, catecholamine and brain natriuretic peptide (BNP) levels are elevated significantly more than in patients with decompensated heart failure after an acute coronary syndrome. Catecholamine levels then start to decline, but remain significantly higher than in patients with acute coronary syndromes even a week after the event. On the other hand, plasma BNP levels decline rapidly, compared to patients with acute coronary events, and this is in parallel with the rapid improvement of the LV systolic function in TC. During the second phase, myocardial stunning occurs as a result of increased catecholamine levels.

3. Proposed mechanisms of Takotsubo syndrome

Plasma catecholamine levels are shown to be closely correlated with TC. In a study by Wittstein et al. [8], plasma catecholamine levels in 13 patients with stress-related myocardial dysfunction were compared with those in 7 patients who presented with acute pulmonary edema after myocardial infarction (Killip class III). The study showed that plasma catecholamine levels (epinephrine, norepinephrine, and dopamine) at presentation were markedly higher among patients with stress-induced cardiomyopathy than among those with Killip class III myocardial infarction. According to the results of this study, patients with stress cardiomyopathy had supraphysiologic levels of plasma catecholamines. Initial plasma levels were several times those of patients with myocardial infarction and remained markedly elevated even a week after the onset of symptoms [8].

The mechanism underlying the association between sympathetic activity and myocardial stunning is unknown.

Increased catecholamine levels result in either direct cardiomyocyte damage through increased calcium levels or in vascular spasm and microvascular dysfunction, which leads to ischemia [5–7]. Abnormal coronary flow in the absence of obstructive disease has recently been reported in patients with stress-related myocardial dysfunction [17]. Increased sympathetic activity and vascular spam also cause an increase in left ventricular afterload adding even more to the pathophysiology of TC [8].

Oxygen-derived free radical circulating levels can be increased by catecholamines and they can cause myocardial injury, which can be attenuated by antioxidants [18]; they can also interfere with sodium and calcium channels, increasing trans-sarcolemmal calcium influx resulting in myocyte dysfunction [19].

Oxidative stress often exaggerates myocardial stunning by affecting calcium homeostasis and causing excitation-contractive uncoupling resulting in myocardial dysfunction [6–8]. The histopathology of the myocardium in this condition differs from that found in ischemic insults and includes a neutrophil-predominant inflammation, contraction band necrosis, and fibrosis [9]. These changes probably reflect calcium cardiotoxicity rather than ischemic necrosis. The pattern of ventricular wall abnormality in TC also points toward a neurally mediated mechanism of cardiac injury [11–13].

One other possibility is ischemia resulting from epicardial coronary arterial spasm. Increased sympathetic tone from mental stress can cause vasoconstriction in patients without coronary disease [20].

A third possible mechanism of catecholamine-mediated myocardial stunning is direct myocyte injury. Elevated catecholamine levels decrease the viability of myocytes through cyclic AMP-mediated calcium overload [21].

4. Nitric oxide: endothelial dysfunction and Takotsubo cardiomyopathy

In 1980, Furchgott and Zawadzki [22] identified the "endothelium-derived relaxing factor" (later recognized as the free gas nitric oxide (NO)) as responsible for the relaxation of vascular smooth muscle cells in response to acetylcholine.

NO is synthesized by the enzyme NO synthase (NOS). This enzyme was first identified and described in the late 1980s. The enzyme NOS catalyzes the biosynthesis of NO through a reaction involving the conversion of L-arginine to L-citruline [23]. NOS is a dimer consisting of two identical monomers, which can be divided into two major domains: the C-terminal reductase and the N-terminal oxygenase domain [24]. It contains binding sites for flavin adenine nucleotide (FAD), nicotinamide adenine dinucleotide phosphate (NADPH) and flavin mono-nucleotide (FMN) in close relation with cytochrome P-450 reductase. The latter binds haem, tetrahydrobiopterin (BH4), and L-arginine, which acts as a substrate.

There are three different NOS isoforms, which differ between them in structure and function [25]. Endothelial NOS (eNOS) and neuronal NOS (nNOS) are Ca^{2+}-dependent enzymes (despite the fact that eNOS can be activated and in an Ca^{2+}-independent manner) [26]. Inducible NOS (iNOS) is only expressed at high levels after induction by cytokines (thus the name inducible) or other inflammatory agents. Its activity is independent of intracellular Ca^{2+} levels. The three NOS isoforms are similar in the way that they have regions of high homology (the oxygenase and the reductase domains) while at the same time each isoform exhibits unique features, which signify their specific functions.

The main source of endothelial NO production is eNOS. Specific properties of eNOS enable the enzyme to perform its specialized functions. These are Ca^{2+} sensitivity and the post-translational modifications, which facilitate sub-cellular localization. These properties enable eNOS to respond not only to hemodynamic forces but to neurohormonal agents as well. There are several factors such as estrogens, hypoxia, and exercise that are known to modify its expression, likely having an impact on cardiovascular function.

4.1 Physiological role of NO: role of NO in vasomotion (vasorelaxation)

As mentioned above, Furchgott and Zawadzki [22] first demonstrated that endothelium reversed the intrinsic constrictive effects of acetylcholine on the vascular smooth muscle through the release of NO. Numerous experimental and clinical studies confirmed that all the arterial endothelium, and to a lesser extent vein endothelium, releases NO. When the endothelium is normal, vasoconstriction is counteracted by the potent vasorelaxing effect of NO. The importance of NO in vasodilation varies between vascular beds and among animal species. Chemical modifications of the guanidino group of L-arginine result in compounds that inhibit NO synthase. NG-nitro-L-arginine (L-NA), NG-monomethyl-L-arginine (L-NMMA), and NG-nitro-L-arginine methyl ester (L-NAME) inhibit the release of NO from endothelial cells, indicating that there is continuous release of NO, which maintains the vasodilator tone.

4.2 The role of L-arginine analogues in eNOS function

ADMA is an amino acid that circulates in plasma, is excreted in urine, and is found in tissues and cells [27–29]. ADMA synthesis involves methylation of arginine residues by protein arginine methyltransferases (PRMTs) [30]. During methylation, either one or two methyl groups are added to the guanidine nitrogens of arginine, which are incorporated into proteins. There are two types of PRMT. Type 1 catalyzes the formation of ADMA and type 2 catalyzes the formation of symmetric dimethylarginine (SDMA) through the methylation of both guanidino nitrogens. Both PRMTs can monomethylate as well. Monomethylation leads to the formation of another asymmetrical form called *NG*-monomethyl-L-arginine (L-NMMA) [31].

The asymmetrical forms (ADMA and L-NMMA) are natural inhibitors of all NOS isoforms, whereas the symmetrical form (SDMA) is not. ADMA and L-NMMA inhibit all three isoforms of NOS [32, 33]. L-NMMA may also uncouple NOS leading to the generation of free radicals and more specific of superoxide [34]. Superoxide formation by this process further results in myocardial injury seen in TC.

Increased sympathetic activity and alterations in NO synthesis attributable to accumulation of ADMA is now recognized as an important mechanism involved in cardiovascular complications [35].

ADMA plasma levels are found to be related to insulin resistance, blood pressure, carotid intima thickness, and age even in healthy individuals, free from cardiovascular disease [36, 37] suggesting that increased ADMA levels are a marker for arteriosclerotic changes.

4.3 Endothelial dysfunction and TC

Increasing data show that endothelial dysfunction is common in patients with TC, which could explain the two of the proposed mechanisms reported at the beginning of this chapter: propensity for epicardial and/or microvascular coronary artery spasm. Indeed, endothelial dysfunction may be a crucial link between myocardial dysfunction seen in TC and stress [38]. Consequently, the reversible LV dysfunction seen in TC may be the result of myocardial stunning due to this ephemeral myocardial ischemia caused by endothelial dysfunction. This mechanism, attenuated by endothelial dysfunction, may also be the cause of high prevalence of TC in postmenopausal women due to estrogen level depletion, which is related to vasomotor abnormalities [39–41].

Under physiological circumstances, estrogens are beneficial for coronary microcirculation. Estrogens have a pivotal role in improving coronary blood flow through endothelium-dependent or independent-mechanisms [41]. Reduced estrogen levels in menopause positively affect endothelial dysfunction and sympathetic drive [40]. Through this effect, postmenopausal estrogen deficiency possibly facilitates the occurrence of TC, especially when emotional stress is in the equation.

Endothelial dysfunction is closely associated to the traditional risk factors for cardiovascular disease. On the other hand, traditional risk factors for cardiovascular disease (smoking, dyslipidemia and hypertension) are present in patients with TC in a non-negligible prevalence [42–44]. In addition, there is growing evidence that patients with TC also have various comorbidities, including neurological, pulmonary, kidney, and liver disease [42], conditions mostly associated with endothelial dysfunction and might therefore constitute a previously unrecognized predisposing factor for TC [45].

5. Conclusion

TC is now a well-recognized syndrome with a very complex pathophysiology. Increased sympathetic activity and plasma catecholamine levels have a pivotal role in the expression of TC. Recent data suggest that endothelial dysfunction and NO depletion are crucial predisposing factors for this syndrome and could be a crucial link between emotional stress and myocardial dysfunction.

Author details

Michael Demosthenous[1], Konstantinos Triantafyllou[2] and Nikolaos Koumallos[2]*

1 Department of Cardiac Surgery, St. Michael's Hospital, University of Toronto, Toronto, Canada

2 Department of Cardiac Surgery, Hippocration General Hospital, Athens, Greece

*Address all correspondence to: koumallosn@yahoo.gr

IntechOpen

References

[1] Akashi YJ, Goldstein DS, Barbaro G, Ueyama T. Takotsubo cardiomyopathy. Circulation. 2008;**118**:2754-2762

[2] Kurowski V, Kaiser A, von Hof K, Killermann DP, Mayer B, Hartmann F, et al. Apical and midventricular transient left ventricular dysfunction syndrome (tako-tsubo cardiomyopathy) frequency, mechanisms, and prognosis. Chest. 2007;**132**:809-816

[3] Schneider B, Athanasiadis A, Schwab J, Pistner W, Gottwald U, Schoeller R, et al. Complications in the clinical course of tako-tsubo cardiomyopathy. International Journal of Cardiology. 2014;**176**:199-205

[4] Hurst RT, Prasad A, Askew JW, Sengupta PP, Tajik AJ. Takotsubo cardiomyopathy: A unique cardiomyopathy with variable ventricular morphology. JACC: Cardiovascular Imaging. 2010;**3**:641-649

[5] Stein AB, Tang XL, Guo Y, Xuan YT, Dawn B, Bolli R. Delayed adaptation of the heart to stress: Late preconditioning. Stroke. 2004;**35**:2676-2679

[6] Ueyama T, Kasamatsu K, Hano T, Yamamoto K, Tsuruo Y, Nishio I. Emotional stress induces transient left ventricular hypocontraction in the rat via activation of cardiac adrenoceptors: A possible animal model of "tako-tsubo" cardiomyopathy. Circulation Journal. 2002;**66**:712-713

[7] Kume T, Kawamoto T, Okura H, Toyota E, Neishi Y, Watanabe N, et al. Local release of catecholamines from the hearts of patients with tako-tsubo-like left ventricular dysfunction. Circulation Journal. 2008;**72**:106-108

[8] Wittstein IS, Thiemann DR, Lima JA, Baughman KL, Schulman SP, Gerstenblith G, et al. Neurohumoral features of myocardial stunning due to sudden emotional stress. The New England Journal of Medicine. 2005;**352**:539-548

[9] Frustaci A, Loperfido F, Gentiloni N, Caldarulo M, Margante E, Russo MA. Catecholamine-induced cardiomyopathy in multiple endocrine neoplasia: A histologic, ultrastructural, and biochemical study. Chest. 1991;**99**:382-385

[10] Ueyama T, Kawabe T, Hano T, Tsuruo Y, Ueda K, Ichinose M, et al. Upregulation of heme oxygenase-1 in an animal model of takotsubo cardiomyopathy. Circulation Journal. 2009;**73**:1141-1146

[11] Pierpont GL, DeMaster EG, Cohn JN. Regional differences in adrenergic function within the left ventricle. The American Journal of Physiology. 1984;**246**:824-829

[12] Simoes MV, Marın-Neto JA, Maciel BC. Variable regional left ventricular dysfunction in takotsubo cardiomyopathy syndrome. Echocardiography. 2007;**24**:893

[13] Kawano H, Okada R, Yano K. Histological study on the distribution of autonomic nerves in the human heart. Heart and Vessels. 2003;**18**:32-39

[14] Cortese B, Robotti S, Puggioni E, Bianchi F, Lupi G, Brignole M. Transient left ventricular apical ballooning syndrome: All that glitters is not apical. Journal of Cardiovascular Medicine. 2007;**8**:934-936

[15] Brandspiegel HZ, Marinchak RA, Rials SJ, Kowey PR. A broken heart. Circulation. 1998;**98**:1349

[16] Gupta S, Goyal P, Idrees S, Aggarwal S, Bajaj D, Mattana J. Association of endocrine conditions

with takotsubo cardiomyopathy: A comprehensive review. Journal of the American Heart Association. 2018 Oct 2;7(19):e009003. DOI: 10.1161/JAHA.118.009003

[17] Bybee KA, Prasad A, Barsness GW, et al. Clinical characteristics and thrombolysis in myocardial infarction frame counts in women with transient left ventricular apical ballooning syndrome. The American Journal of Cardiology. 2004;**94**:343-346

[18] Singal PK, Kapur N, Dhillon KS, Beamish RE, Dhalla NS. Role of free radicals in catecholamine-induced cardiomyopathy. Canadian Journal of Physiology and Pharmacology. 1982;**60**:1390-1397

[19] Bolli R, Marban E. Molecular and cellular mechanisms of myocardial stunning. Physiological Reviews. 1999;**79**:609-634

[20] Lacy CR, Contrada RJ, Robbins ML, et al. Coronary vasoconstriction induced by mental stress (simulated public speaking). The American Journal of Cardiology. 1995;**75**:503-505

[21] Mann DL, Kent RL, Parsons B, Cooper G. Adrenergic effects on the biology of the adult mammalian cardiocyte. Circulation. 1992;**85**:790-804

[22] Furchgott RF, Zawadzki JV. The obligatory role of endothelial cells in the relaxation of arterial smooth muscle by acetylcholine. Nature. 1980;**288**(5789):373-376

[23] Mayer B, Hemmens B. Biosynthesis and action of nitric oxide in mammalian cells. Trends in Biochemical Sciences. 1997;**22**(12):477-481

[24] Hemmens B, Mayer B. Enzymology of nitric oxide synthases. Methods in Molecular Biology. 1998;**100**:1-32

[25] Stuehr DJ. Structure-function aspects in the nitric oxide synthases. Annual Review of Pharmacology and Toxicology. 1997;**37**:339-359

[26] Ayajiki K et al. Intracellular pH and tyrosine phosphorylation but not calcium determine shear stress-induced nitric oxide production in native endothelial cells. Circulation Research. 1996;**78**(5):750-758

[27] van Mourik JA, Romani d WT, Voorberg J. Biogenesis and exocytosis of Weibel-Palade bodies. Histochemistry and Cell Biology. 2002;**117**(2):113-122

[28] McDermott JR. Studies on the catabolism of Ng-methylarginine, Ng, Ng-dimethylarginine and Ng, Ng-dimethylarginine in the rabbit. The Biochemical Journal. 1976;**154**(1):179-184

[29] Cooke JP. Does ADMA cause endothelial dysfunction? Arteriosclerosis, Thrombosis, and Vascular Biology. 2000;**20**(9):2032-2037

[30] Clarke S. Protein methylation. Current Opinion in Cell Biology. 1993;**5**(6):977-983

[31] Vallance P et al. Accumulation of an endogenous inhibitor of nitric oxide synthesis in chronic renal failure. Lancet. 1992;**339**(8793):572-575

[32] MacAllister RJ, Whitley GS, Vallance P. Effects of guanidino and uremic compounds on nitric oxide pathways. Kidney International. 1994;**45**(3):737-742

[33] Olken NM, Marletta MA. NG-methyl-L-arginine functions as an alternate substrate and mechanism-based inhibitor of nitric oxide synthase. Biochemistry. 1993;**32**(37):9677-9685

[34] Pou S et al. Mechanism of superoxide generation by neuronal nitric-oxide synthase. The

Journal of Biological Chemistry. 1999;**274**(14):9573-9580

[35] Tripepi G et al. Inflammation and asymmetric dimethylarginine for predicting death and cardiovascular events in ESRD patients. Clinical Journal of the American Society of Nephrology. 2011;**6**:1714

[36] Perticone F et al. Endothelial dysfunction, ADMA and insulin resistance in essential hypertension. International Journal of Cardiology. 2010;**142**:236

[37] Sydow K et al. Distribution of asymmetric dimethylarginine among 980 healthy, older adults of different ethnicities. Clinical Chemistry. 2010;**56**:111

[38] Naegele M, Flammer AJ, Enseleit F, et al. Endothelial function and sympathetic nervous system activity in patients with takotsubo syndrome. International Journal of Cardiology. 2016;**224**:226-230. DOI: 10.1016/j.ijcard. 2016.09.008

[39] Camici PG, Crea F. Microvascular angina: A women's affair? Circulation. Cardiovascular Imaging. 2015. DOI: 10.1161/CIRCIMAGING. 115.003252

[40] Vitale C, Mendelsohn ME, Rosano GM. Gender differences in the cardiovascular effect of sex hormones. Nature Reviews. Cardiology. 2009;**6**:532-542. DOI: 10.1038/nrcardio.2009.105

[41] Kaski JC. Cardiac syndrome X in women: The role of oestrogen deficiency. Heart. 2006;**92**(Suppl 3): iii5-iii9

[42] Pelliccia F, Parodi G, Greco C, et al. Comorbidities frequency in takotsubo syndrome: An international collaborative systematic review including 1109 patients. The American Journal of Medicine. 2015;**128**(6):654.e11-e19

[43] Templin C, Ghadri JR, Diekmann J, et al. Clinical features and outcomes of takotsubo (stress) cardiomyopathy. The New England Journal of Medicine. 2015;**373**:929-938

[44] Tornvall P, Collste O, Ehrenborg E, Järnbert-Petterson H. A casecontrol study of risk markers and mortality in takotsubo stress cardiomyopathy. Journal of the American College of Cardiology. 2016;**67**:1931-1936. DOI: 10.1016/j.jacc.2016.02.029

[45] Pelliccia F, Greco C, Vitale C, Rosano G, Gaudio C, Kaski JC. Takotsubo syndrome (stress cardiomyopathy): An intriguing clinical condition in search of its identity. The American Journal of Medicine. 2014;**127**:699-704. DOI: 10.1016/j.amjmed.2014.04.004